Diagnostic Ultrasound

Principles, Instruments, and Exercises

Third Edition

Diagnostic Ultrasound

Principles, Instruments, and Exercises

Third Edition

Frederick W. Kremkau, Ph.D.

Professor and Director
Center for Medical Ultrasound
Bowman Gray School of Medicine
Wake Forest University
Winston-Salem, NC

1989

W. B. SAUNDERS COMPANY

Harcourt Brace Jovanovich, Inc.

Philadelphia   London   Toronto
Montreal   Sydney   Tokyo

W.B. SAUNDERS COMPANY
Harcourt Brace Jovanovich, Inc.

The Curtis Center
Independence Square West
Philadelphia, PA 19106

Library of Congress
Cataloging-in-Publication Data

Kremkau, Frederick W.
  Diagnostic ultrasound.

  Previous ed. entered under title.
  Bibliography: p. 352
  1. Diagnosis, Ultrasonic. 2. Diagnosis, Ultrasonic—Problems,
exercises, etc. I. Title.
  RC78.7.U4K745   1989   616.07'543   88–26481
  ISBN 0-7216-2823-0

Designer: Terri Siegel
Production Manager: Peter Faber
Manuscript Editor: Catherine Fix
Illustration Coordinator: Lisa Lambert
Indexer: Linda Van Pelt

Diagnostic Ultrasound: Principles,
Instruments, and Exercises
ISBN   0–7216–2823–0

Last digit is the print number:
9   8   7   6   5   4   3

To Lil and Jonathan

Preface

This book is for sonographers and sonologists who need basic knowledge of the physical principles and instrumentation of diagnostic ultrasound. Its purpose is to explain how diagnostic ultrasound works. It does not describe how to perform diagnostic examinations or how to interpret the results, except in the consideration of artifacts in Chapter 5. Little background in mathematics and physics is assumed. Help in these areas is available in Appendixes C and D, which may be studied before beginning Chapter 1.

Several hundred exercises are provided to check progress, strengthen concepts, and provide practice for registry and specialty-board examinations. Answers are given beginning on page 270. Exercises at the end of each chapter may be used as pretests to determine knowledge in specific subject areas. A comprehensive multiple-choice examination with explanatory referenced answers is given in Appendix E.

An "equals" sign with an asterisk ($\doteq$) indicates that the equation is specifically for soft tissues. An "equals" sign with two asterisks ($\doteq\doteq$) indicates that the equation is specifically for perpendicular incidence at a boundary. A qualitative interpretation is given following each equation.

Superscript numbers refer to citations in the reference list, starting on page 352.

Many statements in this book are simplifications of the actual situation for the sake of brevity.

This third edition contains new and expanded material in the areas of imaging artifacts (Chapter 5), doppler ultrasound (Chapter 6), performance (Chapter 7), and safety (Chapter 7). Gray-scale and color images have been added to enhance the explanation and understanding of principles and concepts.

The word doppler is not capitalized in this book because it is used as an adjective and not as a proper noun. The presentation of attenuation coefficient as equal to approximately one-half the frequency (Section 2.4) is a change from the second edition of this book. This new rule appears to fit the most recent published data.

The author gratefully acknowledges helpful comments and suggestions from instructors and students who have used previous editions of the book. These have resulted in clarifications and improvements in the text and exercises. He thanks Ken Taylor, Jim Sivo, Chris Merritt, Tina Richman, Stan Schwimer, Teresa Jones, and the following companies: Acuson, Advanced Technology Laboratories, General Electric Co. Medical Systems Group, Hewlett-Packard Co. Medical Products Group, Quantum Medical Systems, Inc., ATS Laboratories, Medisonics, Nuclear Associates, Nuclear Enterprises, and Radiation Measurements, Inc., for sharing several of their images and figures that are used throughout the book, as well as Kim Eldridge, Louise Nixon, Jo Patterson, Eric Sullivan, Sharon Hughes, and Sandee Rea for assistance in manuscript preparation and proofreading and Joe Roselli for artwork.

Contents

Chapter 4
Imaging Instruments

Chapter 5
Imaging Artifacts

Chapter 6
Doppler Instruments

Chapter 7
Performance and Safety

Chapter 1

Introduction

There are five reasons for learning the material in this book:

1. to learn how diagnostic ultrasound works
2. to understand and correctly handle artifacts
3. to prepare for instrument performance measurements
4. to be aware of safety and risk considerations
5. to prepare for registry and specialty board examinations.

A survey of over 500 practicing sonographers and sonologists reveals that 88 per cent of physicians and 90 per cent of sonographers agreed with the statement, "Sonographers must know the physics of diagnostic ultrasound."[1]* The inclusion of physical principles in the physician syllabus of the American Institute of Ultrasound in Medicine, in the sonographer syllabus of the Society of Diagnostic Medical Sonographers, in the written examinations of the American Registry of Diagnostic Medical Sonographers and the American Board of Radiology, and in the diagnostic ultrasound educational programs taught around the world attest to the agreement among many in this field on the importance of physics. Ultrasound imaging is not a passive push-button activity. It is an interactive process involving the patient, transducer, instrument, sonographer, and sonologist. Knowledge of the physical principles involved contributes to quality medical care involving diagnostic ultrasound.[2]

In this chapter we consider the question: How does ultrasound image anatomy and measure flow? Ultrasound imaging (sonography) is accomplished with a pulse-echo technique. Pulses of ultrasound (generated by a transducer) are sent into the patient (Fig. 1.1), where they produce

---

* A superscript number refers to a citation in the references section on pages 352–354.

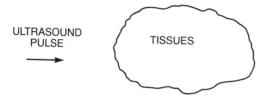

ULTRASOUND
PULSE

TISSUES

Figure 1.1. In diagnostic ultrasound, ultrasound pulses are sent into the tissues to interact with them and obtain information about them. (From Kremkau, F.W.: Ultrasound instrumentation: physical principles. *In* Callen, P.W. [ed.]: Ultrasonography in Obstetrics and Gynecology. Philadelphia, W.B. Saunders Co., 1982. Reprinted with permission.)

echoes at organ boundaries and also within tissues. These echoes return (Fig. 1.2) to the transducer, where they are detected and imaged. Thus, the transducer both generates the ultrasound pulses and detects the returning echoes. The ultrasound instrument processes this information and generates appropriate dots, which form the ultrasound image on the display. The brightness of each dot corresponds to the echo strength. The location of each dot corresponds to the anatomic location of the echo-generating structure. The positional information is determined by knowing the direction of the pulse when it enters the patient and measuring the time for its echo to return to the transducer. From an assumed starting point on the display (usually at the top) the proper location for presenting the echo can then be derived, knowing the direction in which to travel from that starting point to the appropriate distance. The ultrasound pulse and its echo are assumed to travel at 1.54 millimeters per microsecond (μs) in tissue. This means that 13 μs are required for the ultrasound pulse to travel round-trip to a structure located 1 cm away from the transducer (26 μs for 2 cm, 130 μs for 10 cm, and so forth).

Figure 1.3 shows an image of metal rods located at 1, 3, 5, 7, 9, and 11 cm depths in a standard ultrasound test object (American Institute of Ultrasound in Medicine [AIUM] 100-mm test object). Ultrasound instruments use the arrival times of the echoes to locate the rods properly in depth. If one pulse of ultrasound is emitted, one series of dots (one line of information or one scan line) is displayed. From this fact, it is obvious that not all of the ultrasound pulse is reflected back from any inter-

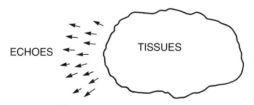

ECHOES

TISSUES

Figure 1.2. Reflected and scattered ultrasound pulses (echoes) return from the tissues providing information useful for imaging, flow measurement, and diagnosis. (From Kremkau, F.W.: Ultrasound instrumentation: physical principles. *In* Callen, P.W. [ed.]: Ultrasonography in Obstetrics and Gynecology. Philadelphia, W.B. Saunders Co., 1982. Reprinted with permission.)

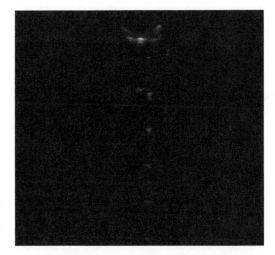

Figure 1.3. An image of metal rods located at 1, 3, 5, 7, 9, and 11 cm depths from the transducer in a standard ultrasound test object. The ultrasound instrument uses the arrival times of the echoes to locate the rods properly in depth. The transducer location is at the top of the image.

face. Rather, a portion of the original pulse will continue on and be reflected back from deeper interfaces. If additional pulses are generated, but each additional pulse has the same path, the same line is displayed over and over again (one repeating scan line). This is demonstrated in Figure 1.4, which shows an image (made with a stationary transducer) of

Figure 1.4. Image of a tissue-equivalent ultrasound phantom made with a stationary transducer (single-repeating scan line).

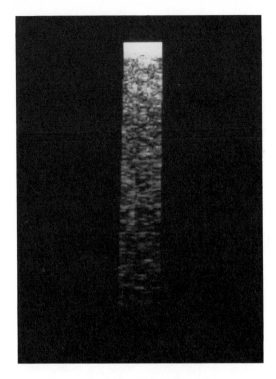

Figure 1.5.   Partial linear scan of
a phantom.

a tissue-equivalent ultrasound phantom. If the process is repeated, but
with different starting points for each subsequent pulse, a cross-sectional
image of the phantom begins to build up. In this case, each pulse travels
in the same direction but starts from a different point. This yields the
parallel scan lines on the display in Figure 1.5. This partial cross-sectional
image of the phantom has been produced with vertical parallel scan lines
that are so close together that they cannot be identified individually.
When the process is complete, a cross-sectional image of the phantom is
produced (Fig. 1.6). The rectangular display resulting from this procedure is often called a linear scan. A second approach to sending
ultrasound pulses through the object to be imaged is shown in Figure 1.7.
Here each pulse originates from the same starting point, but subsequent
pulses go out in slightly different directions from previous ones. This
results in a pie-shaped, windshield-wiper, or sector scan.

There is an unlimited number of scan formats. The linear and sector
scans are the ones used most commonly. Others could be used, but, in
each case, what is required is that ultrasound pulses be sent through all
portions of the cross section that is to be imaged. Each pulse generates a
series of echoes, which results in a series of dots or a scan line on the display. The resulting cross-sectional image is made up of many of these

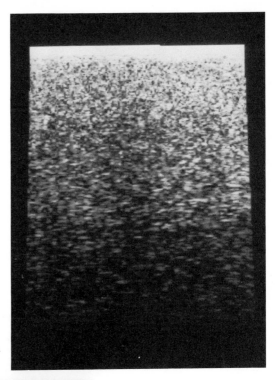

Figure 1.6. Complete linear scan of a phantom.

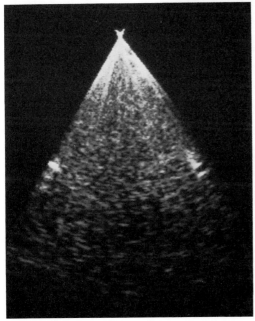

Figure 1.7. Complete sector scan of a phantom.

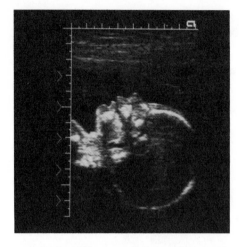

Figure 1.8. Clinical example of a linear scan with its rectangular shape. (Courtesy of Acuson.)

scan lines. The scan format determines the starting points and paths for the individual scan lines according to the starting point and path for each pulse used for generating each scan line. Figures 1.8 and 1.9 are examples of clinical cross-sectional ultrasound images of the linear and sector types, respectively. These are often called "B" scans. This terminology refers to the fact that the images are produced by scanning the ultrasound through the imaged cross section (i.e., sending pulses through all regions of the cross section) and converting echo strength into brightness of each represented echo on the display (thus "B" or brightness scan).

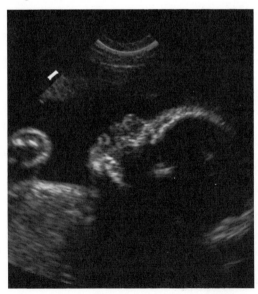

Figure 1.9. Clinical example of a sector scan with its pie-slice shape. (Courtesy of Advanced Technology Laboratories.)

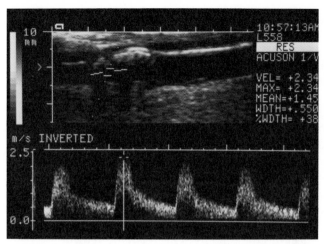

Figure 1.10. Clinical example of a linear scan with doppler blood flow information. (Courtesy of Acuson.)

If an echo-generating structure is moving, the echo will have a different frequency than that of the pulse emitted from the transducer. This is the doppler effect that is put to use primarily in blood-flow measurement. The doppler instrument determines the change in frequency resulting from the motion and converts it into an audible sound or presentation on a display that represents the flow. Figure 1.10 shows the flow in a vessel as a function of time (over several cardiac cycles). Two-dimensional color presentations of flow within vessels in imaged cross-sectional anatomy are shown in Figures 6.13 to 6.16 (Chapter 6).

References 3 to 10 are other sources for the study of diagnostic ultrasound physical principles.

Exercises*

1.1 The diagnostic ultrasound imaging method has two parts:
    1. Sending _____ of _____ into the body.
    2. Using _____ received from the tissues to produce an _____ of internal structures.

1.2 Ultrasound B scans are _____-_____ images of tissue cross sections.

1.3 The brightness of an echo, as presented on the display, represents its _____.

1.4 A linear scan is made up of many _____ scan lines.

---

*Answers to exercises are given beginning on page 270.

1.5 A sector scan is made up of many scan lines with a common _____.

1.6 A linear scan has a _____ shape.

1.7 A sector scan is _____ shaped.

1.8 The _____ effect is used to detect and measure _____ in vessels.

1.9 Motion of an echo-generating structure causes an echo to have a different _____ than the emitted pulse.

1.10 Sonography is accomplished by using a _____-_____ technique. The information of importance in doing this is the _____ from which the echo originated and the _____ of the echo. From these, the echo _____ and _____ on the display are determined.

1.11 In Figure 1.3, how long after the pulse was sent out by the transducer did the echo from the 5-cm rod return?

Chapter 2

Ultrasound

2.1
Introduction

Ultrasound is like the ordinary sound that we hear except that it has a frequency (discussed in the next section) higher than that to which the human hearing system responds. In this chapter we consider the following questions: What is ultrasound and how does it behave? How are continuous and pulsed ultrasound described? How is ultrasound weakened as it travels through tissue? How are echoes generated? The following terms* are discussed in this chapter:

absorption	dB
acoustic	decibel
acoustic propagation properties	density
acoustic variables	duty factor
amplitude	echo
attenuation	effective reflecting area
attenuation coefficient	energy
backscatter	frequency
beam uniformity ratio	half-intensity depth
continuous wave	hertz
continuous-wave mode	impedance
coupling medium	incidence angle
cw	intensity
cycle	intensity reflection coefficient

---

* Terms listed at the beginning of each chapter are defined in the glossary on pages 259–269. Definitions are also given in the summary section of each chapter in which the terms are discussed.

intensity transmission coefficient	rayl
longitudinal wave	reflection
medium	reflection angle
oblique incidence	reflector
particle	refraction
period	scatterer
perpendicular	scattering
perpendicular incidence	sound
propagation	spatial pulse length
propagation speed	specular reflection
pulse	transmission angle
pulse duration	ultrasound
pulse repetition frequency	wave
pulse repetition period	wavelength
pulsed ultrasound	wave variables
range equation	

2.2
Sound

Sound is a wave. A wave is a propagating (traveling) variation in quantities called wave variables. For example, a water wave is a traveling variation in water surface height (the wave variable in this case). Waves carry energy,* not matter, from one place to another. They can also carry information from one place to another, as in the cases of radio, television, radiography, and diagnostic ultrasound. Sound is one particular type of wave. It is a propagating variation in quantities called acoustic variables. These acoustic variables include pressure, density, temperature, and particle motion. A particle is a small portion of the medium through which the sound is traveling. Particles oscillate back and forth as a sound wave travels. Pressure, density, and temperature go through repeating cycles of increase and decrease as the sound wave travels. Unlike light waves and radio waves, sound requires a medium through which to travel; it cannot pass through a vacuum. Sound is a mechanical longitudinal (compressional) wave in which back-and-forth particle motion is parallel to the direction of wave travel.

Sound is described by a few terms common to all waves. These include frequency, period, wavelength, propagation speed, amplitude, and intensity. Frequency, period, amplitude, and intensity are determined

---

*This and other basic physics terms are discussed in Appendix D.

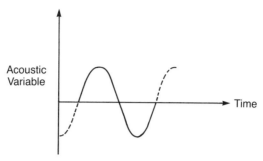

Figure 2.1. One complete variation (cycle) of an acoustic variable (e.g., pressure). This variation repeats as time passes, as indicated by the dashed lines. From Kremkau, F.W.: Basic principles and biological effects of ultrasound. *In* Resnick, M.I., and Sanders, R.C.: Ultrasound in Urology. Baltimore, Williams & Wilkins, 1979. (Reprinted with permission.)

by the sound source. Propagation speed is determined by the medium, and wavelength is determined by both the source and the medium.

Recall that sound is a traveling variation in acoustic variables. Frequency describes how many complete variations (cycles) an acoustic variable goes through in a one second period of time, that is, how many cycles occur in a second. Take pressure as an example of an acoustic variable. Pressure may start at its normal (undisturbed) value, increase to a maximum value, return to normal, decrease to a minimum value, and return to normal (Fig. 2.1). This describes a complete cycle of variation of pressure as an acoustic variable. As a sound wave travels past some point, this cycle is repeated over and over. The number of times that it occurs in 1 second is called the frequency (Fig. 2.2).

Frequency units* include hertz (Hz) and megahertz (MHz). One hertz is one cycle per second or one complete variation per second. *Mega* comes from Greek *megas,* meaning great or large. Specifically, in the metric system of units, it means one million. Therefore, one megahertz is 1,000,000 Hz.

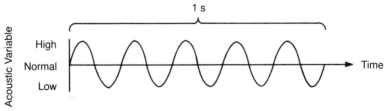

Figure 2.2. Frequency is the number of complete variations (cycles) that an acoustic variable goes through in 1 s. In this figure, five cycles occur each second; the frequency is five cycles per second, or 5 Hz. If five cycles occurred in 1 microsecond (1 μs) (i.e., 5 million cycles in a second), the frequency would be 5 MHz.

---

*Units are discussed in Appendix C.

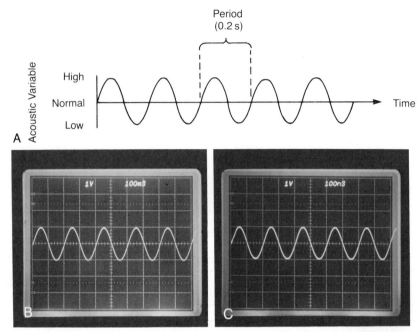

Figure 2.3. Period is the time it takes for one cycle to occur. In (a), each cycle occurs in 0.2 s. The period is 0.2 s, and the frequency is one divided by 0.2 s, or 5 Hz. (b) Photograph of a tracing of a 5-Hz electric voltage. The horizontal scale is 0.1 s per large division. It can be seen that five cycles occur in 1 s. (c) If five cycles occur in 1 μs, the period is 0.2 μs and the frequency is 5 MHz. In this tracing, the horizontal scale is 0.1 μs per division. It can be seen that one cycle occurs in 0.2 μs in this example.

Table C.6 in Appendix C lists unit prefixes. Sound with a frequency of 20,000 Hz or higher is called ultrasound because it is beyond the frequency range of human hearing (approximately 20 Hz to 20,000 Hz). This is analogous to ultraviolet light, which is higher in frequency than human eyes can see (in vision, light frequency is perceived as color; the highest frequency light that we can see is perceived as the color violet). Frequency will be important later when image resolution and imaging depth are considered.

Period is the time that it takes for one cycle to occur (Fig. 2.3). It is equal to one divided by the frequency. Period units include second (s) and microsecond (μs). One microsecond is one millionth of a second (0.000001 s). Period will be important when pulsed ultrasound is considered in the next section. A list of common periods is given in Table 2.1. Period decreases as frequency increases.*

---

*For convenient reference, symbols are compiled in Appendix A and equations in Appendix B. Equations and algebra are discussed in Appendix C. The abbreviations in parentheses represent units appropriate for each quantity (see Appendix C).

Table 2.1
Common Ultrasound Periods and
Wavelengths* in Tissue

Frequency (MHz)	Period (μs)	Wavelength (mm)
1.00	1.00	1.54
2.25	0.44	0.68
3.50	0.29	0.44
5.00	0.20	0.31
7.50	0.13	0.21
10.00	0.10	0.15

*Assume propagation speed of 1.54 mm/μs (1540 m/s).

$$\text{period (μs)} = \frac{1}{\text{frequency (MHz)}} \qquad T = \frac{1}{f}$$

$$\text{frequency} \uparrow \qquad \text{period} \downarrow^*$$

Wavelength is the length of space over which one cycle occurs (Fig. 2.4). If we could stop the sound wave, visualize it, and measure the distance from the beginning to the end of one cycle, the measured distance would be the wavelength. It is really the cycle length, but traditionally it has been called wavelength. Its units include meters (m) and millimeters (mm). One millimeter is one thousandth of a meter (0.001 m). Wavelength will be important when image resolution is considered in Chapter 3.

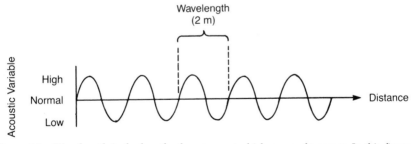

Figure 2.4. Wavelength is the length of space over which one cycle occurs. In this figure, each cycle covers 2 m. The wavelength is 2 m. This figure differs from Figures 2.2 and 2.3 in that the horizontal axis represents distance rather than time. For a propagation speed of 1.54 mm/μs and a frequency of 5 MHz, the wavelength is 0.3 mm.

---

*Beneath each equation in this book is a box containing a qualitative presentation of what it says. The up arrow represents an increase and the down arrow a decrease. Thus, the box related to period contains the statement: as frequency increases, period decreases.

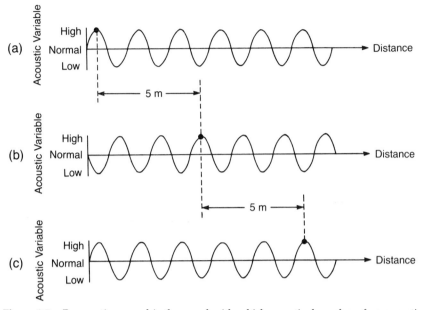

Figure 2.5. Propagation speed is the speed with which a particular value of an acoustic variable moves. The movement of a maximum (identified by the dot) is shown in this figure. Example (b) is 0.5 s after (a). Example (c) is 0.5 s after (b) and 1 s after (a). The maximum (dot) moves 5 m in 0.5 s and 10 m in 1 s. The propagation speed is 10 m/s. The propagation speed in this figure (10 m/s) divided by the frequency in Figure 2.2 (5 Hz) equals the wavelength in Figure 2.4 (2 m). Propagation speeds in tissue are much greater than 10 m/s, averaging 1540 m/s.

Propagation speed* is the speed with which a wave moves through a medium. It is the speed at which a particular value of an acoustic variable moves or with which a cycle moves. An easily identified value of an acoustic variable is its maximum value. The speed with which this maximum value moves through a medium is the propagation speed. (Fig. 2.5). It depends on the medium but not on the frequency.† Wavelength is equal to propagation speed divided by frequency.

$$\text{wavelength (mm)} = \frac{\text{propagation speed (mm/}\mu\text{s)}}{\text{frequency (MHz)}} \qquad \lambda = \frac{c}{f}$$

---

* The word speed is used here rather than velocity because direction of motion is not specified. Velocity is speed with direction of motion specified.

†Propagation speed is not quite independent of frequency. It increases slightly (about 1 m/s/MHz) with frequency in tissues. Because going from 2 to 10 MHz would increase speed by only about 8 m/s (0.5 per cent), this fact can be ignored in imaging.

> frequency ↑   wavelength ↓

An example of the relationship between frequency, wavelength, and propagation speed may be seen by comparing Figures 2.2, 2.4, and 2.5 (see the legend for Fig. 2.5). Propagation speed units include meters per second (m/s) and millimeters per microsecond (mm/μs). One millimeter per microsecond equals 1000 m/s. Wavelength decreases as frequency increases (Table 2.1).

Propagation speed is determined by the density and stiffness (hardness) of the medium. Density is the concentration of matter (mass per unit volume). Stiffness is the resistance of a material to compression. Propagation speed increases if the stiffness is increased or if the density is decreased (a surprising fact for many students). It is generally true that media with higher densities also have higher stiffnesses, but this is not necessarily so. As an illustration, the propagation speed in brass is lower than that in aluminum even though the density of brass is approximately three times that of aluminum.

In general, propagation speeds are low through gases, are higher through liquids, and are the highest through solids. This increasing sequence is not caused by the increasing density (which produces a decreasing propagation speed) but by the increasing stiffness. This is because the stiffness differences between gases, liquids, and solids are larger than the density differences. The average propagation speed in soft tissues (i.e., excluding bone) is 1540 m/s or 1.54 mm/μs. Values for specific tissues are given in Table 2.2. In lung (which contains gas), the propagation speed is lower than in other soft tissues, generally in the range of 0.3 to 1.2 mm/μs.[*] Goss and coworkers[12] give propagation speed values for various tissues. Values for fat (about 1.44 mm/μs) are significantly lower (by about 6 percent) than the soft tissue average. Propagation speed is important because imaging instruments make use of it in generating the display. This is discussed in Chapters 1 and 4. Using the average propagation speed for soft tissue, wavelength is as follows.[†]

For soft tissues:

$$\text{wavelength (mm)} \overset{*}{=} \frac{1.54}{\text{frequency (MHz)}} \qquad \lambda \overset{*}{=} \frac{1.54}{f}$$

---

[*] In Section 2.4 we see that ultrasound does not penetrate lung or bone well, so that these differing propagation speeds are normally not of concern.

[†]An equals sign with an asterisk indicates that the equation is specifically for soft tissues.

Table 2.2
Propagation Speeds in
Soft Tissues[11,12]

Tissue	Propagation Speed (mm/μs)
Fat	1.44
Brain	1.51
Liver	1.56
Kidney	1.56
Muscle	1.57
Soft tissue average	1.54

A list of common wavelengths is given in Table 2.1.

Impedance is equal to density multiplied by propagation speed.* It will be important for the discussion of reflections later in this chapter. Its

$$\text{impedance (rayl)} = \text{density (kg/m}^3) \times \text{propagation speed (m/s)} \qquad z = pc$$

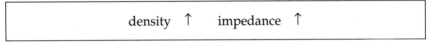

density ↑   impedance ↑

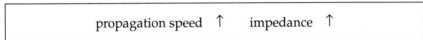

propagation speed ↑   impedance ↑

unit is the rayl. Impedance is determined by the density and stiffness of a medium. It increases if the density is increased or if the stiffness is increased. Recall that propagation speed also depends on density and stiffness, but in a different way. Impedance does not depend on frequency (see footnote on frequency dependence of propagation speed on page 14).

Typical values for frequency, period, wavelength, propagation speed, and impedance are given in Table 2.7 in Section 2.6.

---

*The impedance described here is the characteristic acoustic impedance, which is defined as density times propagation speed. The impedance used in Section 2.5 is *not* the characteristic impedance, but rather the specific acoustic impedance, which is defined as pressure divided by particle velocity. The two impedances are equal for a plane (nondiverging or converging) wave in a nonattenuating medium.

Exercises

2.2.1 A wave is a traveling variation in quantities called _____.

2.2.2 Sound is a traveling variation in quantities called _____.

2.2.3 Ultrasound is sound with a frequency of _____ Hz or higher.

2.2.4 Acoustic variables include _____, _____, _____, and _____.

2.2.5 Which of the following frequencies are in the ultrasound range? (More than one correct answer.)
   a. 15 Hz
   b. 15,000 Hz
   c. 15 MHz
   d. 30,000 Hz
   e. 0.04 MHz

2.2.6 Which of the following are acoustic variables? (More than one correct answer.)
   a. pressure
   b. frequency
   c. propagation speed
   d. period
   e. particle motion

2.2.7 Frequency is a measure of how many _____ an acoustic variable goes through in a second.

2.2.8 The unit of frequency is the _____, which is abbreviated _____.

2.2.9 Period is the _____ that it takes for one cycle to occur.

2.2.10 Period is one divided by _____.

2.2.11 Wavelength is the length of _____ over which one cycle occurs.

2.2.12 Propagation speed is the speed with which a _____ moves through a medium.

2.2.13 Wavelength is equal to _____ divided by _____.

2.2.14 Propagation speed is determined by the _____ and _____ of a medium.

2.2.15 Propagation speed increases if
   a. density is increased
   b. density is decreased
   c. stiffness is increased
   d. a and c
   e. b and c

2.2.16 The average propagation speed in soft tissues is _____ m/s or _____ mm/µs.

2.2.17 Propagation speed is determined by
  a. frequency
  b. amplitude
  c. wavelength
  d. period
  e. medium

2.2.18 Place the following in order of increasing sound propagation speed:
  a. gas
  b. solid
  c. liquid

2.2.19 The wavelength of 1-MHz ultrasound in soft tissues is _____ mm.

2.2.20 Wavelength in soft tissues _____ as frequency increases.

2.2.21 It takes _____ µs for ultrasound to travel 1.54 cm in soft tissue.

2.2.22 Propagation speed in bone is _____ than in soft tissues.

2.2.23 Sound travels fastest in
  a. air
  b. helium
  c. water
  d. iron
  e. a vacuum

2.2.24 Solids have higher propagation speeds than liquids because they have higher
  a. density
  b. stiffness

2.2.25 The propagation speeds through mercury and fat are approximately the same, even though the density of mercury is approximately 15 times that of fat. This means that the stiffness of mercury must be much _____ than that of fat.

2.2.26 Sound is a _____ _____ wave.

2.2.27 If propagation speed is doubled (a different medium) and frequency is held constant, the wavelength is _____ .

2.2.28 If wavelength in a given medium at a given frequency is 2 mm and the frequency is doubled, the wavelength becomes _____ mm.

2.2.29 If frequency in soft tissue is doubled, propagation speed is _____ .

2.2.30 Waves carry _____ from one place to another. They can also carry _____ from one place to another.

2.2.31 From given values for propagation speed and frequency, which of the following can be calculated?
  a. amplitude
  b. period
  c. wavelength
  d. a and b
  e. b and c

2.2.32 If two media have the same stiffness but different densities, the one with the higher density will have the higher propagation speed. True or false?

2.2.33 If two media have the same density but different stiffnesses, the one with the higher stiffness will have the higher propagation speed. True or false?

2.2.34 If the density is 1000 kg/m^3 and the propagation speed is 1.54 mm/μs, the impedance is _____ rayls.

2.2.35 If two media have the same stiffness but different densities, the one with the higher density will have the higher impedance. True or false?

2.2.36 If two media have the same density but different stiffnesses, the one with the higher stiffness will have the higher impedance. True or false?

2.2.37 Impedance is _____ multiplied by _____ _____.

2.2.38 What are the periods and frequencies shown in Figure 2.6?

2.2.39 If the wavelength in Figure 2.6(a) is 0.154 mm, the propagation speed is _____ mm/μs.

2.2.40 If the propagation speed is 1.54 mm/μs, the wavelength in Figure 2.6(b) is _____ mm.

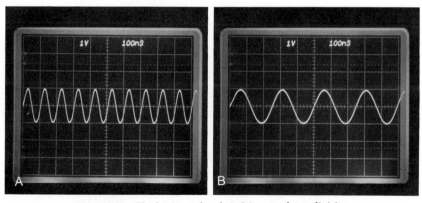

Figure 2.6. The horizontal scale is 0.1 μs per large division.

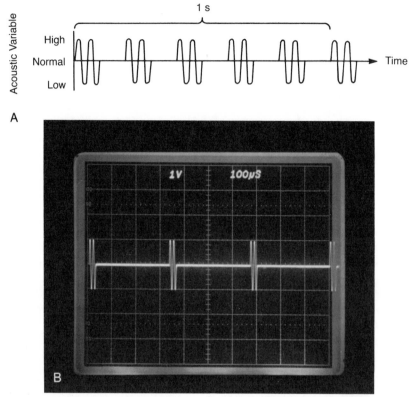

Figure 2.7. Pulse repetition frequency is the number of pulses occurring in 1 s. In (a), five pulses (containing two cycles each) occur in 1 s; thus, the pulse repetition frequency is 5 Hz. In (b), a photograph of a tracing of electric voltage, three pulses occur in 1 ms; thus, the pulse repetition frequency is 3 kHz. Horizontal scale is 0.1 ms per large division.

2.3
Pulsed Ultrasound

The terms discussed earlier (frequency, period, wavelength, and propagation speed) describe a continuous wave (cw). For diagnostic ultrasound imaging, continuous-wave sound is not used. Instead, short pulses of sound are used. This is called pulsed ultrasound. It is produced by applying electrical pulses to the transducer (see Chapter 3). Ultrasound pulses are described by some additional parameters that have not yet been introduced.

Pulse repetition frequency is the number of pulses occurring in 1 second (Fig. 2.7). Its units include the hertz (Hz) and kilohertz (kHz). One kilohertz is 1000 Hz.

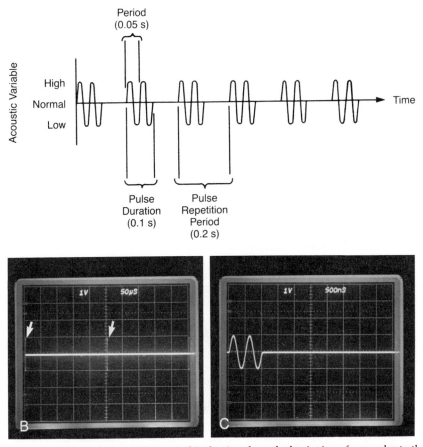

Figure 2.8. The pulse repetition period is the time from the beginning of one pulse to the beginning of the next. In (a), the pulse repetition period is 0.2 s. Therefore, the pulse repetition frequency is 5 Hz. Pulse duration is the time that it takes for one pulse to occur. It is equal to the period times the number of cycles in the pulse. In (a), pulse duration is 0.1 s. Because two cycles occur in a 0.1-s pulse in this figure, the period is 0.05 s, and the frequency is 20 Hz. The duty factor is the fraction of time that the sound is on. It is pulse duration divided by pulse repetition period. The duty factor in (a) is 0.5 (the sound is on half the time). In (b), a photograph of a tracing of electric voltage, the pulse repetition period is 0.25 ms (pulse repetition frequency is 4 kHz), the period is 0.5 μs as shown expanded in (c), and the pulse duration is 1 μs. Duty factor is, therefore, 0.004 or 0.4 per cent.

The pulse repetition period is the time from the beginning of one pulse to the beginning of the next (Fig. 2.8). Its units include seconds (s) and milliseconds (ms). One millisecond is one thousandth of a second (0.001 s). The pulse repetition period is one divided by pulse repetition frequency.

$$\text{pulse repetition period (ms)} = \frac{1}{\text{pulse repetition frequency (kHz)}}$$

$$PRP = \frac{1}{PRF}$$

pulse repetition frequency ↑   pulse repetition period ↓

Pulse duration is the time that it takes for a pulse to occur (Fig. 2.8)[*] It is equal to the period times the number of cycles in the pulse. Its units include seconds (s) and microseconds (µs).

pulse duration (µs) = number of cycles in pulse x period (µs) $PD = nT$

$$= \frac{\text{number of cycles in pulse}}{\text{frequency (MHz)}} \qquad PD = \frac{n}{f}$$

period ↑   pulse duration ↑

number of cycles in the pulse ↑   pulse duration ↑

frequency ↑   pulse duration ↓

The second equation is derived from the first by substituting one divided by frequency for period. Pulse duration decreases if the number of cycles is decreased or if frequency is increased.

Duty factor is the fraction of time that sound (in the form of pulses)

---

[*] Pulse duration must be specified by some definition of where in time to start and stop. For example, a 10-dB pulse duration is the time during which the pulse intensity (Section 2.4) is one tenth or greater of the maximum occurring in the pulse.

is on. It is calculated by dividing the pulse duration by the pulse repetition period. The duty factor is unitless. It will be important when intensities are discussed in Section 2.4.

$$\text{duty factor} = \frac{\text{pulse duration (µs)}}{\text{pulse repetition period (ms) x 1000}} \qquad DF = \frac{PD}{PRP \times 1000}$$

$$\text{duty factor} = \frac{\text{pulse duration (µs)} \times \text{pulse repetition frequency (kHz)}}{1000} \qquad DF = \frac{PD \times PRF}{1000}$$

pulse duration ↑   duty factor ↑

pulse repetition period ↑   duty factor ↓

pulse repetition frequency ↑   duty factor ↑

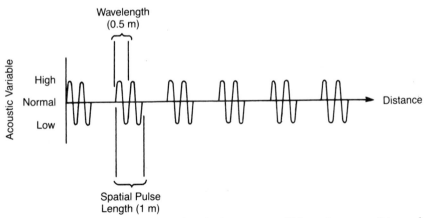

Figure 2.9. Spatial pulse length is the length of space over which a pulse occurs. It is equal to wavelength times the number of cycles in the pulse. In this figure, wavelength is 0.5 m; there are two cycles in each pulse; and spatial pulse length is 0.5 times 2, or 1 m. This figure differs from Figures 2.7(a) and 2.8(a) in that the horizontal axis represents distance rather than time.

The second equation is derived from the first by substituting one divided by pulse repetition frequency for pulse repetition period. By multiplying the duty factor by 100, the result is expressed in per cent.

Spatial pulse length is the length of space over which a pulse occurs (Fig. 2.9). It is equal to the wavelength times the number of cycles in the pulse. Its units include meters (m) and millimeters (mm). It will be an important quantity when axial resolution is discussed in Section 3.5.

spatial pulse length (mm) = number of cycles in pulse x wavelength (mm)	$SPL = n\lambda$
spatial pulse length (mm) = $\dfrac{\text{number of cycles in pulse} \times \text{propagation speed (mm/}\mu s)}{\text{frequency (MHz)}}$	$SPL = \dfrac{nc}{f}$
For soft tissues: spatial pulse length (mm) $\overset{*}{=} \dfrac{\text{number of cycles in pulse} \times 1.54}{\text{frequency (MHz)}}$	$SPL \overset{*}{=} \dfrac{n \times 1.54}{f}$

wavelength ↑	spatial pulse length ↑

number of cycles in the pulse ↑	spatial pulse length ↑

frequency ↑	spatial pulse length ↓

The second equation is derived from the first by substituting propagation speed divided by frequency for wavelength.

The propagation speed for pulses is the same as that for continuous waves in a given medium. Frequency within pulses is not the same as that for continuous waves. A continuous wave may be described by a single frequency. Pulses contain frequencies in addition to the specified (operating) frequency. This is discussed in Section 3.2. Pulses have many frequencies present (see Fig. 3.6 in Chapter 3). The shorter the pulse, the greater the bandwidth. The dominant frequency present in the pulse is close to or equal to the frequency for the unpulsed (cw) wave. For pulses, frequency gives the number of cycles per second, assuming continuous waves (even though this assumption is not correct for pulsed ultrasound). Therefore, 1-MHz pulsed ultrasound with a duty factor of 0.1 per cent will have only 1000 cycles per second (because the quiet time between pulses eliminates 99.9 per cent of the cycles), even though the frequency implies that there are 1 million cycles per second.

Typical values for pulse repetition frequency, pulse repetition period, pulse duration, duty factor, and spatial pulse length are given in Table 2.7 in Section 2.6.

Exercises

2.3.1 The abbreviation cw stands for _____ _____.

2.3.2 Pulsed ultrasound is ultrasound in the form of repeated short _____.

2.3.3 Pulse repetition frequency is the number of _____ occurring in 1 s.

2.3.4 Pulsed ultrasound is produced by applying electrical _____ to the transducer.

2.3.5 The pulse repetition _____ is the time from the beginning of one pulse to the beginning of the next.

2.3.6 The pulse repetition period is one _____ the pulse repetition frequency.

2.3.7 Pulse duration is the _____ for a pulse to occur.

2.3.8 Spatial pulse length is the _____ of _____ over which a pulse occurs.

2.3.9 _____ _____ is the fraction of time that pulsed ultrasound is actually on.

2.3.10 Pulse duration equals the number of the cycles in the pulse times _____.

2.3.11 Spatial pulse length equals the number of cycles in the pulse times _____.

2.3.12 The duty factor of continuous-wave sound is _____.

2.3.13 If the wavelength is 2 mm, the spatial pulse length for a three-cycle pulse is _____ mm.

2.3.14 The spatial pulse length in soft tissue for a four-cycle pulse of frequency 3 MHz is _____ mm.

2.3.15 The pulse duration in soft tissue for a four-cycle pulse of frequency 3 MHz is _____ μs.

2.3.16 For a 1-kHz pulse repetition frequency, the pulse repetition period is _____ ms.

2.3.17 For Exercises 2.3.15 and 2.3.16 together, the duty factor is
_____.

2.3.18 How many cycles are there in 1 s of continuous-wave 5-MHz
ultrasound?
a. 5
b. 500
c. 5000
d. 5,000,000
e. none of the above

2.3.19 How many cycles are there in 1 s of pulsed 5-MHZ ultrasound
with duty factor of 0.001?
a. 5
b. 500
c. 5000
d. 5,000,000
e. none of the above

2.3.20 In Exercise 2.3.19, how many cycles were eliminated by pulsing?
a. 100 per cent
b. 99.9 per cent
c. 99 per cent
d. 50 per cent
e. 1 per cent

2.3.21 For pulsed ultrasound, the duty factor is always _____
_____ one.

2.4
Attenuation

The rate at which cycles occur in time (frequency), the time required
for each cycle (period), the space over which a cycle occurs (wavelength),
and the speed at which the cycles move (propagation speed) have been
described. The magnitude of the variations will now be considered. This
will give some idea of the strength of the sound. Amplitude and intensity
are the parameters that are relevant here. They would be measures of
how loud the sound would be if it could be heard. Of course, it cannot be
heard because it is ultrasound.

Amplitude is the maximum variation that occurs in an acoustic variable. It is the maximum value minus the normal (undisturbed) value
(Fig. 2.10). Amplitude is given in units appropriate for the acoustic variable considered.

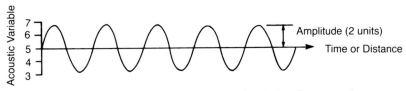

Figure 2.10. Amplitude is the maximum amount of variation that occurs in an acoustic variable. It is equal to the maximum value of the variable minus the normal (undisturbed) value. In this figure, the amplitude is seven (maximum value) minus five (normal value); the amplitude is two units.

Intensity is the power in a wave divided by the area over which the power is spread (Fig. 2.11).

$$\text{intensity (W/cm}^2) = \frac{\text{power (W)}}{\text{area (cm}^2)} \qquad I = \frac{P}{A}$$

power ↑   intensity ↑

area ↑   intensity ↓

Power is discussed in Appendix D. Power units include watts (W) and milliwatts (mW). If the total power across a sound beam is divided by the beam area, the spatial average intensity is calculated. This is discussed later in this section. Sound beams and beam area are discussed in Section 3.3. Beam area units are centimeters squared (cm²). Intensity

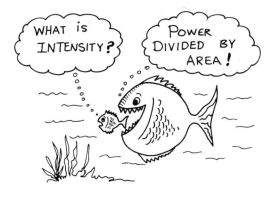

Figure 2.11. Intensity is the power in a sound wave divided by the area over which the power is spread.

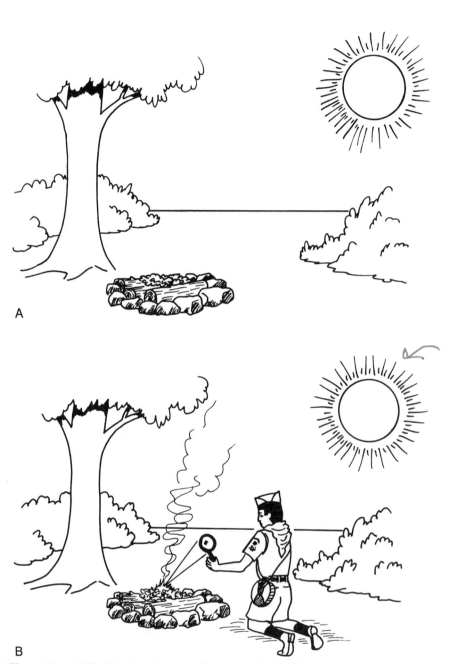

A

B

Figure 2.12. (a) Sunlight does not normally ignite a fire. (b) With focusing of the sunlight (increased intensity), ignition can occur.

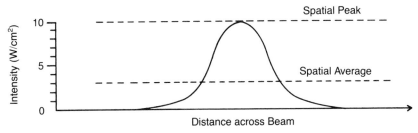

Figure 2.13. Intensity is a function of distance across the beam. In this figure, the spatial peak intensity (at the beam center) is 10 W/cm^2, the spatial average is 3 W/cm^2, and the beam uniformity ratio is 3.3. In addition to varying across the beam, intensity varies along the direction of the beam.

units include watts per centimeter squared (W/cm^2) and others listed in Table C.7 (Appendix C). Intensity is an important parameter in describing the sound that is produced and received by diagnostic instruments (Chapter 4) and in discussing bioeffects and safety (Chapter 7). It may be illustrated by analogy with sunlight incident on dry leaves (Fig. 2.12). Sunlight will not normally ignite the leaves, but if the same power is concentrated into a small area (increased intensity) by focusing with a magnifying glass, the leaves can be ignited. An effect is therefore produced by increasing the intensity even though the power remains the same.

It will be seen in Section 3.3 that beam area is determined in part by the size and operating frequency of the sound source chosen. For a given beam power, intensity will be determined by the beam area resulting from the choice of sound source.

Intensity is proportional to the amplitude squared. Thus, if amplitude is doubled, intensity is quadrupled. If amplitude is halved, intensity is quartered.

Because intensity is not uniform across a sound beam (Fig. 2.13) and, in the case of pulsed ultrasound, is not uniform in time (Fig. 2.14),

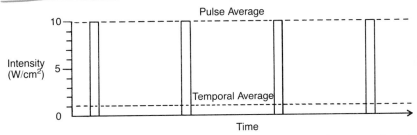

Figure 2.14. Intensity as a function of time for pulsed ultrasound. Pulse average intensity (10 W/cm^2) is the intensity when the sound is actually on. Temporal average intensity (1 W/cm^2) is the intensity that results when this is averaged over time. In this figure, the duty factor is 0.1.

several intensities are used. For spatial considerations either the spatial peak (SP) or the spatial average (SA) value may be used. These are related by the beam uniformity ratio, which is defined as the spatial peak intensity divided by the spatial average intensity.

---

spatial average intensity (W/cm²) =

$$\frac{\text{spatial peak intensity (W/cm}^2)}{\text{beam uniformity ratio}}$$ $I_{SA} = \dfrac{I_{SP}}{BUR}$

---

beam uniformity ratio ↑   spatial average intensity ↓

---

spatial peak intensity ↑   spatial average intensity ↑

$BUR = \dfrac{I_{SP}}{I_{SA}}$

For temporal (time) considerations, the temporal average (TA) value or pulse average (PA) value may be used. These are related by the duty factor.

$DF = \dfrac{I_{TA}}{I_{PA}}$

---

temporal average intensity (W/cm²) =
duty factor x pulse average intensity (W/cm²) $I_{TA} = DF \times I_{PA}$

---

duty factor ↑   temporal average intensity ↑

---

pulse average intensity ↑   temporal average intensity ↑

If the sound is continuous instead of pulsed, the duty factor is equal to one, and the pulse average and temporal average intensities are equal to each other. The four intensities resulting from spatial and temporal considerations are spatial average–temporal average (SATA) intensity, spatial peak–temporal average (SPTA) intensity, spatial average–pulse average (SAPA) intensity, and spatial peak–pulse average (SPPA) intensity.

duty factor: length of time u/s is actually on

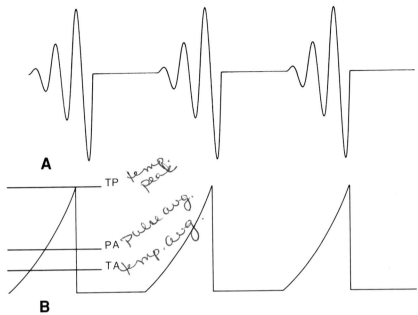

Figure 2.15 (a) Ultrasound pulses used in imaging. These pulses have cycles of differing amplitudes. They are produced by electrical shock excitation of a damped transducer (see Chapter 3 and Figure 3.5 for details). (b) Intensity of the pulses in (a). TP = temporal pulse, PA = pulse average, and TA = temporal average intensities.

The pulses shown in Figures 2.7 and 2.14 have constant amplitude and intensity during each pulse. Although pulses used in doppler ultrasound are similar to these, pulses used in ultrasound imaging are typically like that shown in Figure 2.15. In this case the peak intensity occurring within each pulse is called the temporal peak (TP) intensity. The intensity averaged over the pulse duration is called the pulse average (PA) intensity. For constant amplitude pulses, such as those in Figures 2.7 and 2.14, temporal peak and pulse average intensities are the same. Combining spatial considerations with the temporal peak intensity yields spatial average–temporal peak (SATP) and spatial peak–temporal peak (SPTP) values.

Example 2.4.1

The SATA intensity is 1 mW/cm^2, the beam uniformity ratio is 10, and the duty factor is 0.002. Calculate SPTA, SAPA, and SPPA intensities.

$$\text{SPTA intensity} = \text{SATA intensity} \times \text{beam uniformity ratio}$$
$$= 1 \times 10 = 10 \text{ mW/cm}^2$$

$$\text{SAPA intensity} = \frac{\text{SATA intensity}}{\text{duty factor}}$$

$$= \frac{1}{0.002} = 500 \text{ mW/cm}^2$$

$$\text{SPPA intensity} = \frac{\text{SATA intensity} \times \text{beam uniformity ratio}}{\text{duty factor}}$$

$$= \frac{1 \times 10}{0.002} = 5000 \text{ mW/cm}^2 = 5 \text{ W/cm}^2$$

SATA intensity is the lowest of the four, and SPPA intensity is the highest. SPTA and SAPA intensities have intermediate values, with SAPA normally being the greater of the two. For pulses as in Figure 2.15, SPTP intensity is higher than SPPA intensity.

Example 2.4.2

The SPTP and SPPA intensities of pulsed ultrasound are 60 and 20 W/cm^2, respectively. Calculate the other four intensities given that the beam uniformity ratio is 20 and the duty factor is 0.001.

$$\text{SAPA intensity} = \frac{\text{SPPA intensity}}{\text{beam uniformity ratio}}$$

$$= \frac{20}{20} = 1 \text{ W/cm}^2$$

$$\text{SPTA intensity} = \text{SPPA intensity} \times \text{duty factor}$$

$$= 20 \times 0.001 = 20 \text{ mW/cm}^2$$

$$\text{SATA intensity} = \frac{\text{SPPA intensity} \times \text{duty factor}}{\text{beam uniformity ratio}}$$

$$= \frac{20 \times 0.001}{20} = 1 \text{ mW/cm}^2$$

$$\text{SATP intensity} = \frac{\text{SPTP intensity}}{\text{beam uniformity ratio}}$$

$$= \frac{60}{20} = 3 \, \text{W}/\text{cm}^2$$

The terms discussed previously (frequency, period, wavelength, propagation speed, amplitude, and intensity) describe sound waves. Another term, attenuation, needs to be defined before sound reflection is considered in the next section. It is important to understand attenuation because it must be compensated for by the diagnostic instrument (Section 4.3).

For an unfocused beam (beams and focus are discussed in Chapter 3) in any medium such as tissue, amplitude and intensity will decrease as the sound travels through the medium. This reduction in amplitude and intensity as sound travels is called attenuation (Fig. 2.16). It encompasses absorption (conversion of sound to heat), reflection, and scattering (Section 2.5). Absorption is normally the dominant contribution to attenuation in soft tissues. Attenuation units are decibels (dB). The attenuation coefficient is the attenuation per unit length of sound travel. Its units are decibels per centimeter (dB/cm). See Appendix C for a discussion of decibels. The longer the path over which the sound travels, the greater the attenuation.

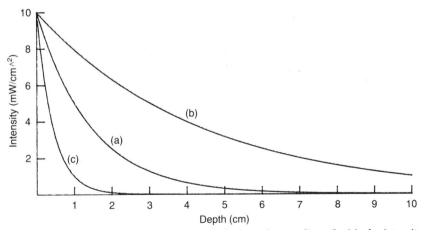

Figure 2.16. Attenuation of sound as it travels through a medium. In (a), the intensity decreases by 50 per cent for each 1 cm of travel. This corresponds to an attenuation coefficient of 3 dB/cm. In (b), attenuation coefficient is 1 dB/cm and in (c) it is 10 dB/cm.

Table 2.3
Attenuation Coefficients in
Tissue at 1 MHz

Tissue	Attenuation Coefficient (dB/cm)
Fat	0.6
Brain	0.6
Liver	0.7
Kidney	0.9
Muscle	1.0
Heart	1.1

attenuation (dB) = attenuation coefficient (dB/cm) $a = a_c l$
                    x path length (cm)

attenuation coefficient   ↑   attenuation   ↑

path length   ↑   attenuation   ↑

The attenuation coefficient increases with increasing frequency. Persons who live in apartments or dormitories experience this fact when they hear mostly the bass notes through the wall from a neighbor's sound system. For soft tissues, attenuation coefficients are given in Table 2.3. A simple proportional approximation is that soft tissue, on the average, has 0.5 dB of attenuation per centimeter for each megahertz of frequency (Table 2.4). Therefore, the average attenuation coefficient in

Table 2.4
Average Attenuation Coefficients in Tissue

Frequency (MHz)	Average Attenuation Coefficient for Soft Tissue (dB/cm)	Intensity Reduction in 1-cm Path (%)	Intensity Reduction in 10-cm Path (%)
1.00	0.5	11	68
2.25	1.1	22	92
3.50	1.8	34	98
5.00	2.5	44	99.7
7.50	3.8	58	99.98
10.00	5.0	68	99.999

decibels per centimeter for soft tissues is approximately equal to one half the frequency in megahertz.* In order to calculate the attenuation in decibels, simply multiply half the frequency in megahertz (which is approximately equal to the attenuation coefficient in dB/cm) by the path length in centimeters, and the result is the attenuation in decibels.

For soft tissues:

$$\text{attenuation coefficient (dB/cm)} \stackrel{*}{=} \frac{1}{2} \times \text{frequency (MHz)} \qquad a_c \stackrel{*}{=} \frac{1}{2} f$$

$$\text{attenuation (dB)} \stackrel{*}{=} \frac{1}{2} \times \text{frequency (MHz)} \times \text{path length (cm)} \qquad a \stackrel{*}{=} \frac{1}{2} fl$$

---

frequency ↑   attenuation coefficient ↑

---

frequency ↑   attenuation ↑

The intensity ratio corresponding to that number of decibels may be obtained from Table C.2 in Appendix C. This ratio is equal to the fraction of the intensity (at the beginning of the path) that remains at the end of the path. If the intensity at the beginning is known, the intensity at the end may be found by multiplying by the intensity ratio. A summary of this four-step process is:

1. One half times frequency (MHz) yields attenuation coefficient (dB/cm).
2. Attenuation coefficient (dB/cm) times path length (cm) yields attenuation (dB).
3. Find the intensity ratio in Table C.2 for the decibel value calculated in step 2.
4. The intensity ratio times the intensity at the start of the path equals the intensity at the end of the path.

---

*This rule (Table 2.4), although a good description of attenuation values experienced in normal ultrasound-imaging practice, yields attenuation values that are lower than those found in laboratory measurements (Table 2.3).

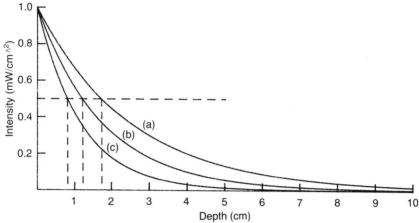

Figure 2.17. Intensity versus depth in tissue for (a) 3.5 MHz, (b) 5.0 MHz, and (c) 7.5 MHz in soft tissues. Half-intensity depth (1.7, 1.2, and 0.8 cm, respectively) is indicated for each.

Example 2.4.3

If 4-MHz ultrasound at 10 mW/cm² SATA intensity is applied to a soft tissue surface, what is the SATA intensity 1.5 cm into the tissue? One half the frequency yields an attenuation coefficient of 2 dB/cm. Attenuation coefficient (2 dB/cm) multiplied by the path length (1.5 cm) is equal to 3 dB. The attenuation is 3 dB. From Table C.2 (Appendix C) it can be found that 3 dB corresponds to an intensity ratio of 0.5. Thus, 50 per cent of the intensity remains after the sound travels through this path. The intensity ratio (0.5) times the SATA intensity at the beginning of the path (10 mW/cm²) gives the SATA intensity at the end of the path (5 mW/cm²).

Attenuation is higher in lung than in other soft tissues. In bone it is

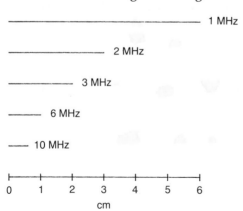

Figure 2.18. Half-intensity depth for several frequencies in soft tissues. Half-intensity depth decreases as frequency increases.

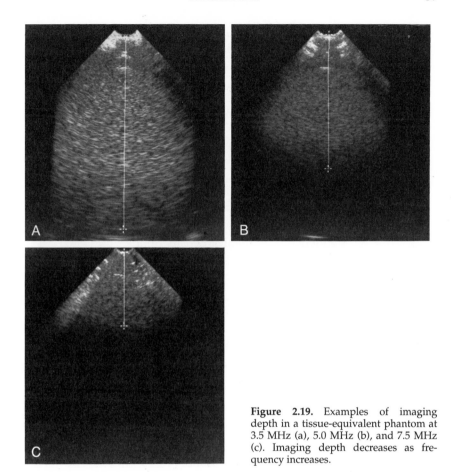

Figure 2.19. Examples of imaging depth in a tissue-equivalent phantom at 3.5 MHz (a), 5.0 MHz (b), and 7.5 MHz (c). Imaging depth decreases as frequency increases.

higher than in soft tissues. Lung and bone attenuations are not proportionally dependent on frequency. Therefore, the four-step process just described cannot be used for them (specifically, step one fails).

A practical consequence of attenuation is that it limits the depth at which images can be obtained. A useful parameter related to this is the half-intensity depth. This is defined as the depth at which intensity is reduced to 50 per cent (3 dB) of its original value (Fig. 2.17). It therefore is also the distance over which 50 per cent of the original intensity is lost. The half-intensity depth decreases as frequency increases (Fig. 2.18). It is useful when considering to what depths in a tissue imaging may be accomplished. However, half-intensity depth does not imply that imaging cannot be performed beyond this depth. It normally can. The two are related, so that if half-intensity depth decreases (for example, because of an increase in frequency), imaging depth also decreases (Fig. 2.19). Table 2.5 lists half-intensity depths for various frequencies in soft tissue.

$$\text{half-intensity depth (cm)} = \frac{3}{\text{attenuation coefficient (dB/cm)}} \qquad D = \frac{3}{a_c}$$

For soft tissues:

$$\text{half-intensity depth} \stackrel{*}{=} \frac{6}{\text{frequency (MHz)}} \qquad D \stackrel{*}{=} \frac{6}{f}$$

frequency ↑   half-intensity depth ↓

The second equation is derived from the first by substituting one half the frequency for attenuation coefficient.

Exercises

2.4.1 Amplitude is the maximum _____ that occurs in an acoustic variable.

2.4.2 Intensity is the _____ in a wave divided by _____.

2.4.3 The unit for intensity is _____.

2.4.4 Intensity is proportional to the square of _____.

2.4.5 If power is doubled and area remains unchanged, intensity is _____.

Table 2.5
Common Values for Various
Diagnostic Ultrasound Terms

Frequency (MHz)	Wavelength (mm)	Attenuation Coefficient (dB/cm)	Half-Intensity Depth (cm)
1.00	1.54	0.5	6.0
2.25	0.68	1.1	2.7
3.50	0.44	1.8	1.7
5.00	0.31	2.5	1.2
7.50	0.21	3.8	0.8
10.0	0.15	5.0	0.6

2.4.6 If area is doubled and power remains unchanged, intensity is _____.

2.4.7 If both power and area are doubled, intensity is _____.

2.4.8 If amplitude is doubled, intensity is _____.

2.4.9 If a sound beam has a power of 10 mW and a beam area of 2 cm², the spatial average intensity is _____ mW/cm².

2.4.10 The beam uniformity ratio is the spatial _____ intensity divided by the spatial _____ intensity.

2.4.11 The duty factor is equal to temporal _____ intensity divided by _____ average intensity.

2.4.12 Which of the following intensities are equal for continuous-wave sound?
a. spatial peak and spatial average
b. temporal peak and temporal average
c. spatial peak and temporal average
d. spatial average and temporal average
e. none of the above

2.4.13 If the SATA intensity is 1 mW/cm², the beam uniformity ratio is 3, and the duty factor is 0.001, calculate the following intensities:
a. SPTA: _____ mW/cm²
b. SAPA: _____ W/cm²
c. SPPA: _____ W/cm²

2.4.14 If pulsed ultrasound is on 50 per cent of the time (duty factor = 0.5) and pulse average intensity is 4 mW/cm², temporal average intensity is _____ mW/cm².

2.4.15 If the maximum value of an acoustic variable is 10 units and the normal (undisturbed) value is 7 units, the amplitude is _____ units. The minimum value of the acoustic variable is _____.

2.4.16 Attenuation is the reduction in _____ and _____ as a wave travels through a medium.

2.4.17 Attenuation consists of _____, _____, and _____.

2.4.18 The attenuation coefficient is attenuation per unit _____ of sound travel.

2.4.19 The attenuation and attenuation coefficient are given in the units _____ and _____, respectively.

2.4.20 For soft tissues, there is approximately _____ dB of attenuation per centimeter for each megahertz of frequency.

2.4.21 For soft tissues, the attenuation coefficient at 3 MHz is approximately _____.

2.4.22 The attenuation coefficient in soft tissue _____ as frequency increases.

2.4.23 For soft tissue, if frequency is doubled, attenuation is _____; if path length is doubled, attenuation is _____; if both frequency and path length are doubled, attenuation is _____.

2.4.24 If frequency is doubled and path length is hàlved, attenuation is _____.

2.4.25 Absorption is the conversion of _____ to _____.

2.4.26 Can the absorption be greater than the attenuation in a given medium at a given frequency? _____.

2.4.27 Is attenuation in bone higher or lower than in soft tissue? _____.

2.4.28 For average soft tissue, the attenuation is such that for each 1.5 cm traveled, a 4-MHz sound intensity is reduced by _____ per cent and the half-intensity depth is _____ cm. For 1 cm and 6 MHz, the reduction is _____ per cent and the half-intensity depth is _____ cm.

2.4.29 The half-intensity depth for soft tissue at 10 MHz is _____ cm.

2.4.30 The attenuation coefficient for soft tissue at 5 MHz is _____ dB/cm.

2.4.31 The half-intensity depth in soft tissue is three divided by _____ or six divided by _____.

2.4.32 The half-intensity depth _____ as frequency increases.

2.4.33 If the intensity of 4-MHz ultrasound entering soft tissue is 2 W/cm^2, the intensity at a depth of 4 cm is _____ W/cm^2. The half-intensity depth is _____ cm.

2.4.34 If the intensity of 40-MHz ultrasound entering soft tissue is 2 W/cm^2, the intensity at a depth of 4 cm is _____ W/cm^2.

2.4.35 The half-intensity depth in soft tissues at 7.5 MHz is _____ cm.
   a. 0.6
   b. 0.7
   c. 0.8
   d. 0.9
   e. 1.0

2.5
Echoes

Thus far in this chapter, the propagation of ultrasound through homogeneous media has been considered. The usefulness of ultrasound as an imaging tool is primarily the result of reflection and scattering at organ boundaries and scattering within heterogeneous tissues. These phenomena will be considered in this section.

Perpendicular incidence (sometimes called normal incidence) occurs when the direction of travel of the ultrasound is perpendicular to the boundary between two media (Fig. 2.20). If the incidence is not perpendicular, it is called oblique incidence.

When there is perpendicular incidence, the incident sound may be reflected or transmitted, or both (Fig. 2.21). Reflected sound travels through medium one in a direction opposite to the incident sound (i.e., the reflected sound returns to the sound source). Transmitted sound moves through medium two in the same direction as the incident sound.

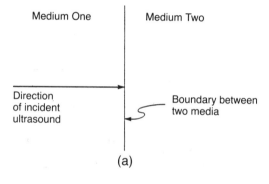

(a)

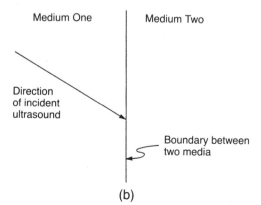

Figure 2.20. Perpendicular incidence (a) and oblique incidence (b) at a boundary between two media.

(b)

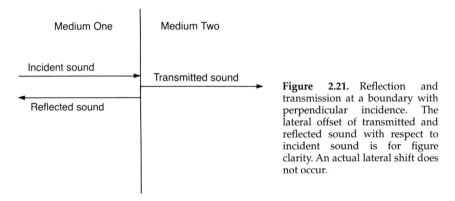

Figure 2.21. Reflection and transmission at a boundary with perpendicular incidence. The lateral offset of transmitted and reflected sound with respect to incident sound is for figure clarity. An actual lateral shift does not occur.

The intensities of the reflected sound and transmitted sound depend on the incident intensity and the impedances of the media.

The reflected intensity divided by the incident intensity is called the intensity reflection coefficient. The transmitted intensity divided by the incident intensity is called the intensity transmission coefficient. These coefficients give the fractions of incident sound intensity that are reflected and transmitted, respectively. They must add up to one in order to

---

With perpendicular incidence*:

$$\text{intensity reflection coefficient} = \frac{\text{reflected intensity (W/cm}^2)}{\text{incident intensity (W/cm}^2)}$$

$$\overset{**}{=} \left[\frac{\text{medium two impedance} - \text{medium one impedance}}{\text{medium two impedance} + \text{medium one impedance}} \right]^2$$

$$\text{IRC} = \frac{I_r}{I_i} \overset{**}{=} \left[\frac{z_2 - z_1}{z_2 + z_1} \right]^2$$

$$\text{intensity transmission coefficient} = \frac{\text{transmitted intensity (W/cm}^2)}{\text{incident intensity (W/cm}^2)}$$

$$\overset{**}{=} 1 - \text{intensity reflection coefficient}$$

$$\text{ITC} = \frac{I_t}{I_i} \overset{**}{=} 1 - \text{IRC}$$

---

*An equation with two asterisks above the equals sign is specifically for perpendicular incidence.

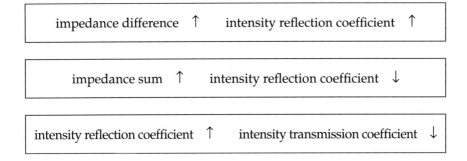

| impedance difference ↑ | intensity reflection coefficient ↑ |

| impedance sum ↑ | intensity reflection coefficient ↓ |

| intensity reflection coefficient ↑ | intensity transmission coefficient ↓ |

account for all the incident sound intensity (what is not reflected must be transmitted).

It can be seen that, for perpendicular incidence, if the media impedances are the same, there is no reflected sound, and transmitted intensity is equal to incident intensity. If there is no reflection, the media impedances are equal. It can also be seen that the reflected and transmitted intensities depend not only on the (subtraction) difference between the media impedances but also on their sum (compare Exercises 2.5.4 and 2.5.5, in which the impedance differences are the same but the answers are different, and compare Exercises 2.5.4 and 2.5.6, in which impedance differences are different but the answers are the same).

Recall that impedance is density times propagation speed (Section 2.2). For perpendicular incidence, a reflection is generated at a boundary if the impedances are different. A reflection may be generated when the densities are the same if the propagation speeds are different (see Exercise 2.5.10). On the other hand, no reflection may be generated even when the densities are different (see Exercise 2.5.11). If there is a large difference between the impedances, there will be almost total reflection (intensity reflection coefficient close to one, intensity transmission coefficient close to zero). An example of this is an air–soft tissue boundary (see Exercise 2.5.17). For this reason, a coupling medium (an oil or a gel) is used to provide a good sound path from the source to the skin during the diagnostic use of ultrasound.

Example
2.5.1

For impedances of 40 and 60 rayls, calculate the intensity reflection and transmission coefficients.

$$\text{intensity reflection coefficient} = \left[\frac{60-40}{60+40}\right]^2 = \left[\frac{20}{100}\right]^2 = 0.2^2 = 0.2 \times 0.2 = 0.04$$

$$\text{intensity transmission coefficient} = 1 - 0.04 = 0.96$$

The intensity reflection coefficient can be expressed as 4 per cent and the intensity transmission coefficient as 96 per cent. The sum of the two coefficients is 100 per cent, i.e., all of the incident intensity must be either reflected or transmitted.

If the incident intensity is known, the reflected and transmitted intensities can be calculated by multiplying the incident intensity by the intensity reflection coefficient and the intensity transmission coefficient, respectively.

Example 2.5.2

For Example 2.5.1, if the incident intensity is 10 mW/cm^2 calculate the reflected and transmitted intensities.

From Example 2.5.1, the intensity reflection and transmission coefficients are 0.04 and 0.96, respectively.

$$\text{reflected intensity} = 10 \times 0.04 = 0.4 \text{ mW/cm}^2$$

$$\text{transmitted intensity} = 10 \times 0.96 = 9.6 \text{ mW/cm}^2$$

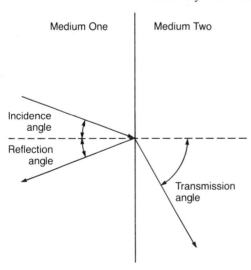

Figure 2.22. Reflection and transmission at a boundary with oblique incidence. Incidence and reflection angles are equal. The transmission angle depends on the incidence angle and the media propagation speeds.

These coefficients give the fraction of the incident intensity that is reflected or transmitted. By multiplying the coefficients by 100, these fractions are expressed in per cent. They must always add up to 1 (or 100 per cent). In Example 2.5.2, all of the incident intensity is accounted for (4 per cent reflected, 96 per cent transmitted, for a total of 100 per cent).

Oblique incidence occurs when the direction of travel of the incident ultrasound is not perpendicular to the boundary between two media (Fig. 2.20). This is the common situation in diagnostic ultrasound. The direction of travel with respect to the boundary is given by the incidence angle (for perpendicular incidence, the incidence angle is zero). The reflected and transmitted directions are given by the reflection angle and transmission angle, respectively (Fig. 2.22). They are related as follows:[*]

---

reflection angle (degrees) = incidence angle (degrees) $\theta_r = \theta_i$

transmission angle (degrees) = incidence angle (degrees) x

$$\left[\frac{\text{medium two propagation speed (mm/\mu s)}}{\text{medium one propagation speed (mm/\mu s)}} \right] \qquad \theta_t = \theta_i \left[\frac{c_2}{c_1} \right]$$

The second equation is the refraction equation. A change in direction of sound (transmission angle unequal to incidence angle) when crossing a boundary is called refraction (Latin, to turn aside). The transmission angle is greater than the incidence angle if the propagation speed through medium two is greater than the propagation speed through medium one (Fig. 2.23[a]). There is no refraction if the propagation speeds are equal (Fig. 2.23[b]) or if the incidence angle is zero (perpendicular incidence). Refraction is important because, when it occurs, lateral position errors occur on an image. This is discussed further in Section 5.3.

---

[*]The second equation is an approximation. The correct form is:

---

sine of transmission angle (degrees) =

$$\sin \theta_t = (\sin \theta_i) \frac{c_2}{c_1}$$

sine of incidence angle (degrees) x

$$\frac{\text{medium two propagation speed (mm/\mu s)}}{\text{medium one propagation speed (mm/\mu s)}}$$

For small incidence angles, the difference is not significant.

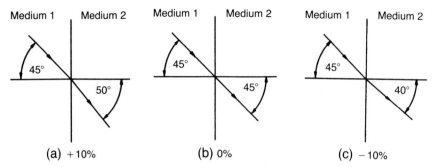

Figure 2.23. Transmission angles for an incidence angle of 45 degrees and propagation speeds through medium two (a) 10 per cent greater than, (b) equal to, and (c) 10 per cent less than propagation speed through medium one.

Example 2.5.3

If the incidence angle is 20 degrees, the propagation speed in medium one is 1.6 mm/μs and the propagation speed in medium two is 1.4 mm/μs, calculate the reflection and transmission angles.

$$\text{reflection angle} = \text{incidence angle} = 20 \text{ degrees}$$

$$\text{transmission angle} = \text{incidence angle} \times \left(\frac{\text{speed}_2}{\text{speed}_1}\right)$$

$$= 20\left(\frac{1.4}{1.6}\right) = 17.5 \text{ degrees}$$

Refraction occurs with light as well as with sound. It is the principle on which lenses operate. It is also the cause of distortion when viewing objects in a fish bowl. As with sound, when light crosses a boundary obliquely, where a change in light speed occurs, the direction of the light travel changes.

Expressions for calculating oblique reflection and transmission coefficients are more complicated than those that apply when there is perpendicular incidence, and they are not given here. For given media, the reflection coefficient for oblique incidence may be smaller than, equal to, or greater than that for normal incidence, depending on incidence angle. If the propagation speeds through the media are the same, the intensity reflection coefficient is the same as that for perpendicular incidence and is independent of incidence angle. For oblique incidence it is possible for a reflection to occur even if the media have equal impedances. This will occur if the propagation speeds are different. Conversely, it

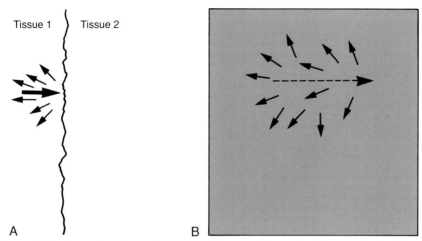

Figure 2.24. A sound pulse may be scattered by a rough boundary between tissues (A) or from within tissues owing to their heterogeneous character (B). (From Kremkau, F.W.: Ultrasound instrumentation: Physical principles. *In* Callen, P.W. [ed.]: Ultrasonography in Obstetrics and Gynecology. Philadelphia, W.B. Saunders, 1982. Reprinted with permission.)

is possible that no reflection will occur even when the media impedances are different. Therefore, absence of reflection with oblique incidence does not necessarily mean that the media impedances are equal (as it does with perpendicular incidence).

It is sometimes stated by authors that reflection amplitude decreases with increasing incidence angle. Whether this is true or not depends on the densities and propagation speeds involved. It is possible, with certain values of propagation speed and density, for the reflection amplitude to increase, decrease, or remain constant as angle increases. The reflection amplitude may pass through a minimum and then increase or start at zero (equal impedances) and increase.

Previously in this section, it was assumed that wavelength is small compared with the boundary dimensions and with boundary roughness. The resulting reflections are called specular reflections. If, on the other hand, the boundary dimensions are comparable to or small compared with the wavelength, or if the boundary is not smooth (surface irregularities comparable in size to the wavelength), the incident sound will be scattered (diffused). Scattering is the redirection of sound in many directions by rough surfaces or by heterogeneous media, such as (cellular) tissues, or particle suspensions, such as blood (Fig. 2.24). These cases are analogous to light in which specular (Latin, mirror) reflections occur at mirrors. For a rougher surface, such as a white wall, although virtually all the light is reflected (that is why the wall is white) the image

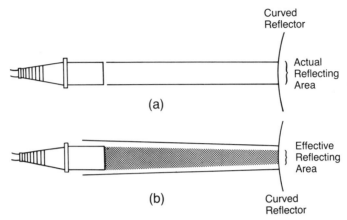

Figure 2.25. A curved reflector. (a) Incident sound on reflecting area. (b) Reflected sound from reflecting area. Only part of this reflected sound (shaded portion from the effective reflecting area) returns to the transducer. The remainder misses the transducer and continues on. The effective reflecting area is smaller than the actual reflecting area.

is not observed (as in a mirror) because the light is scattered at the surface and mixed up as it travels back to the viewer's eyes. When light passes through a suspension of water droplets in air (fog), it is scattered as well. This limits the viewer's ability to see through fog. Although scattering inhibits vision (we cannot see ourselves reflected in a wall and we cannot see well through fog), it is of great benefit in ultrasound imaging. Here the desire is to see the "wall" (tissue interface), not a reflection of "oneself" (the sound source). There is also a desire to see the "fog" (tissue parenchyma), not just objects beyond it.

Backscatter (sound scattered back in the direction from which it originally came) intensities from rough surfaces and heterogeneous media vary with frequency and scatterer size. They may be comparable to or less than specular reflection intensities from tissue boundaries. Normally, scatter intensities are much less than boundary specular reflection intensities. The roughness of a tissue boundary or heterogeneity of a medium (such as tissue) effectively increases as frequency is increased (increased backscatter). This is because wavelength decreases as frequency increases, thus making wavelength smaller relative to roughness or scatterer dimensions. This is why the sky is blue. Light is scattered more strongly by particles suspended in the atmosphere for higher frequencies (low frequency light is red, high frequency light is blue).

The intensity received by the sound source from specular reflections is highly angle-dependent. Scattering from boundaries helps to make echo reception less dependent on incidence angle. Because diagnostic ultrasound is confined to beams (Section 3.3), there are conditions in which all or part of the reflected sound may not return to the transducer

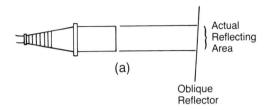

(a)

Oblique
Reflector

Figure 2.26. An oblique reflector. (a) Incident sound on reflecting area. (b) Reflected sound from reflecting area. Only part of this reflected sound (shaded portion) returns to the transducer from the effective reflecting area. The remainder misses the transducer and continues on. The effective reflecting area is smaller than the actual reflecting area.

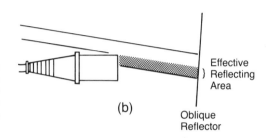

(b)

Oblique
Reflector

and thus will be missed. Figures 2.25 and 2.26 show examples of simple situations in which this occurs. The effective reflecting area, the area that reflects sound that is received by the transducer, is smaller than the actual reflecting areas in these cases. Therefore, reflector orientation and shape may reduce the amount of beam area received by the transducer. A curved reflector can produce a reflection low in amplitude because some of the reflection is missed by the transducer. Oblique reflection can produce a reflection low in amplitude, or the reflection may be completely missed by the transducer. This problem is reduced by reflector roughness, which adds backscatter to specular reflection. Increasing the frequency effectively increases the reflector roughness.

Scattering, then, permits ultrasound imaging of tissue boundaries that are not necessarily perpendicular to the direction of the incident sound. It also allows imaging of tissue parenchyma as well as organ boundaries. Scattering is relatively independent of the direction of the incident sound and therefore is more characteristic of the scatterers. Reflections from smooth boundaries depend not only on the acoustic properties at the boundaries but also on the angles involved.

Because the ultrasound pulse encounters several scatterers at any point in its travel, several echoes are generated simultaneously. These may arrive at the transducer in such a way that they reinforce (constructive interference) or partially or totally cancel (destructive interference) each other. This results in a displayed dot pattern that does not directly represent scatterers, but rather represents an interference pattern of the scatterer distribution scanned. This phenomenon is called acoustic speckle. It is analogous to the speckle phenomenon observed with lasers.

Now that sound propagation, reflection, and scattering have been considered, a very important factor for pulse-echo diagnostic ultrasound, the range equation, can be studied. The approach in pulse-echo diagnostic ultrasound is (1) to generate short pulses of sound that travel through the body, producing reflections (echoes) that travel back to the source, and (2) to detect and display the returning echoes. The method that the instruments use to properly position the echo on the display is described in Chapter 4. The two items of information required are (1) the direction from which the echo came (which is assumed to be the direction in which the source is pointed), and (2) the distance to the boundary (reflector or scatterer) where the echo was produced. The distance is calculated from the range (distance to reflector) equation:

---

distance to reflector (mm) =

$$d = \frac{1}{2}ct$$

$\frac{1}{2}$[propagation speed (mm/µs) x pulse round-trip time (µs)]

---

round-trip time ↑   reflector distance ↑

---

propagation speed ↑   round-trip time ↓

To obtain the distance from the source to the reflector, the propagation speed in the intervening medium must be known or assumed, and the pulse round-trip time must be measured. The reason that the factor ½ appears is that the round-trip time is the time for the pulse to travel to the reflector and return. However, only the distance *to* the reflector is desired. The soft tissue average propagation speed (1.54 mm/µs) is usually assumed in using the range equation (unless another speed is given). For this case:

For soft tissues:

distance to reflector (mm) $\stackrel{*}{=}$ 0.77 x pulse round-trip time (µs) $d \stackrel{*}{=} 0.77t$

Table 2.6
Pulse Round-Trip
Travel Time for
Various Reflector Depths

Depth (cm)	Travel Time (μs)
0.5	6.5
1	13
2	26
3	39
4	52
5	65
10	130
15	195
20	260

This equation was derived from the range equation by substituting 1.54 mm/μs for the speed and dividing by 2 to get 0.77. If the pulse round-trip time is 13 μs, substitution in the equation above yields a reflector distance of 10 mm (1 cm). This leads to the well-known 13 μs/cm rule. That is, pulse round-trip travel time is 13 μs for each centimeter of distance from source to reflector (Table 2.6). The foregoing equation can be converted to the following by recognizing that $0.77 = \frac{1}{1.3}$ and changing mm to cm:

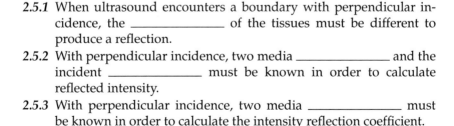

$$\text{distance to reflector (cm)} \stackrel{*}{=} \frac{\text{pulse round-trip time (μs)}}{13} \qquad d \stackrel{*}{=} \frac{t}{13}$$

Exercises

2.5.1 When ultrasound encounters a boundary with perpendicular incidence, the _____ of the tissues must be different to produce a reflection.

2.5.2 With perpendicular incidence, two media _____ and the incident _____ must be known in order to calculate reflected intensity.

2.5.3 With perpendicular incidence, two media _____ must be known in order to calculate the intensity reflection coefficient.

2.5.4 For an incident intensity of 2 mW/cm^2 and impedances of 49 and 51 rayls, the reflected intensity is _____ mW/cm^2, and the transmitted intensity is _____ mW/cm^2.

2.5.5 For an incident intensity of 2 mW/cm^2 and impedances of 99 and 101 rayls, the reflected and transmitted intensities are _____ and _____ mW/cm^2.

2.5.6 For an incident intensity of 2 mW/cm^2 and impedances of 98 and 102 rayls, the reflected and the transmitted intensities are _____ and _____ mW/cm^2.

2.5.7 For an incident intensity of 5 mW/cm^2 and impedances of 45 and 55 rayls, the intensity reflection coefficient is _____ or _____ per cent.

2.5.8 For impedances of 45 and 55 rayls, the intensity transmission coefficient is _____ or _____ per cent.

2.5.9 For impedances of 45 and 55 rayls, the intensity reflection coefficient is _____ dB.

2.5.10 Given the following:
incident intensity = 1 mW/cm^2
medium one:
   density = 1.0 kg/m^3
   propagation speed = 1350 m/s
medium two:
   density = 1.0 kg/m^3
   propagation speed: 1650 m/s
The reflected intensity is _____ mW/cm^2.

2.5.11 Given the following:
incident intensity = 5 mW/cm^2
medium one:
   density = 1.00 kg/m^3
   propagation speed = 1515 m/s
medium two:
   density = 1.01 kg/m^3
   propagation speed = 1500 m/s
The reflected intensity is _____ mW/cm^2.

2.5.12 Given the following:
incident intensity = 5 mW/cm^2
medium one impedance = 2 rayls
medium two impedance = 0 rayls
The reflected and transmitted intensities are _____ and _____ mW/cm^2.

2.5.13 If the impedances of the media are equal, there is no reflection. True or false?

2.5.14 If the densities of the media are equal, there is no reflection. True or false?

2.5.15 If propagation speeds of the media are equal, there is no reflection. True or false?

2.5.16 The intensity reflection and transmission coefficients depend on whether the sound is traveling from medium one into medium two or vice versa. True or false?

2.5.17 The intensity reflection coefficient at a boundary between soft tissue (impedance 1,630,000 rayls) and air (impedance 400 rayls) is _____.

2.5.18 A coupling medium is used to eliminate _____ between the sound source and the skin, thus eliminating a strong _____ at the air-skin boundary.

2.5.19 The intensity reflection coefficient at a boundary between fat (impedance 1,380,000 rayls) and muscle (impedance 1,700,000 rayls) is _____.

2.5.20 The intensity reflection coefficient at a boundary between soft tissue (impedance 1,630,000 rayls) and bone (impedance 7,800,000 rayls) is _____.

2.5.21 With perpendicular incidence, the reflected intensity depends on
   a. density difference
   b. acoustic impedance difference
   c. acoustic impedance sum
   d. both b and c
   e. both a and b

2.5.22 Refraction is a change in _____ of sound when it crosses a boundary.

2.5.23 If the propagation speed through medium two is larger than the propagation speed through medium one, the transmission angle will be _____ the incidence angle, and the reflection angle will be _____ the incidence angle.

2.5.24 If the propagation speed through medium two is smaller than the propagation speed through medium one, the transmission angle will be _____ the incidence angle, and the reflection angle will be _____ the incidence angle.

2.5.25 If the propagation speed through medium two is equal to the propagation speed through medium one, the transmission angle will be _____ the incidence angle, and the reflection angle will be _____ the incidence angle.

2.5.26 If the incidence angle is 30 degrees, the propagation speed through medium one is 1 mm/µs and the propagation speed through medium two is 0.7 mm/µs, the reflection angle is

_____ degrees and the transmission angle is _____ degrees.

2.5.27 If the incidence angle is 30 degrees, the propagation speed through medium one is 1 mm/μs and the propagation speed through medium two is 1 mm/μs, the reflection angle is _____ degrees and the transmission angle is _____ degrees.

2.5.28 If the incidence angle is 30 degrees and the propagation speed through medium two is 30 per cent higher than the propagation speed through medium one, the reflection angle is _____ degrees and the transmission angle is _____ degrees.

2.5.29 Given the following:

incidence angle = 20 degrees
incident intensity = 5 mW/cm^2
propagation speed through medium one = 1.5 mm/μs
impedance of medium one = 8 rayls
propagation speed through medium two = 1.5 mm/μs
impedance of medium two = 12 rayls

the reflection coefficient is ____.

2.5.30 Given the following:

incidence angle = 20 degrees
incident intensity = 5 mW/cm^2
transmission angle = 20 degrees
impedance of medium one = 8 rayls
impedance of medium two = 12 rayls

the reflected intensity is _____ mW/cm^2.

2.5.31 Under what two conditions does refraction not occur?

a. _____
b. _____

2.5.32 Under what condition is the reflection coefficient not dependent on incidence angle?

2.5.33 When ultrasound encounters a boundary with oblique incidence, either _____ or _____ _____ must change in order to generate a reflection.

2.5.34 The low speed of sound in fat is a source of image degradation because of refraction. If the incidence angle at a boundary between fat (1440 m/s) and kidney (1560 m/s) is 30 degrees, the transmission angle is _____ degrees.

2.5.35 For Exercise 2.5.34, the lateral shift of the sound path 5 cm beyond the boundary because of refraction is _____ mm. Proceed as follows: The difference between the incidence and transmission angles is 2 degrees. The tangent of 2 degrees is 0.0349. The tangent multiplied by the distance (5 cm) yields the lateral shift.

2.5.36 Redirection of sound in many directions as it encounters rough media junctions or particle suspensions (heterogeneous media) is called _____.

2.5.37 With specular reflection, wavelength is small compared with boundary dimensions. True or false?

2.5.38 Scattering occurs when boundary dimensions are large compared with wavelength or when the boundary is smooth. True or false?

2.5.39 As frequency increases, backscatter strength
a. increases
b. decreases
c. does not change
d. refracts
e. infarcts

2.5.40 Backscatter helps make echo reception less dependent on incidence angle. True or false?

2.5.41 As frequency increases, specular reflections
a. increase
b. decrease
c. do not change
d. refract
e. infarct

2.5.42 The approach in pulse-echo ultrasound is (1) to generate _____ of sound that travel through the body, producing _____ that travel back to the source, and (2) to detect and _____ the returning echoes.

2.5.43 To calculate the distance to a reflector, the _____ _____ and the pulse round-trip _____ must be known.

2.5.44 If the propagation speed is 1.6 mm/μs and the pulse round-trip time is 5 μs, the distance to the reflector is _____ mm.

2.5.45 If the propagation speed is 1.4 mm/μs and the time for a pulse to travel to the reflector is 5 μs, the distance to the reflector is _____ mm.

2.5.46 When the pulse round-trip time is 10 μs, the distance to a reflector in soft tissue is _____ mm.

2.5.47 When the pulse round-trip time is 13 μs, the distance to a reflector in soft tissue is _____ cm.

2.5.48 When the pulse round-trip time is 39 μs, the distance to a reflector in soft tissue is _____ mm.

2.5.49 When the pulse round-trip time is 130 μs, the distance to a reflector in soft tissue is _____ mm.

2.6
Review

Ultrasound is sound (a wave of traveling acoustic variables: pressure, density, temperature, and particle motion) of frequency greater than 20 kHz. It is described by frequency, period, wavelength, propagation speed, amplitude, intensity, and attenuation. Pulsed ultrasound is described by additional terms: pulse repetition frequency, pulse repetition period, pulse duration, duty factor, and spatial pulse length. Propagation speed and impedance are characteristics of the medium that are determined by density and stiffness. Attenuation increases with frequency and path length. Half-intensity depth decreases with increasing frequency. Six intensities (SATA, SPTA, SAPA, SPPA, SATP, and SPTP) are used to describe pulsed ultrasound. The soft tissue propagation speed is 1.54 mm/μs, and the attenuation coefficient is 0.5 dB/cm for each megahertz of frequency. Table 2.7 gives typical values for several parameters of diagnostic ultrasound. Table 2.8 indicates how various parameters change with frequency.

When, with perpendicular incidence, sound encounters boundaries between media with different impedances, part of the sound is reflected and part is transmitted. If the two media have the same impedance, there is no reflection. With oblique incidence, the sound is refracted at a boundary between media where propagation speeds are different. Incidence and reflection angles are always equal. For oblique incidence

Table 2.7
Diagnostic Ultrasound Parameters in Tissue

Parameter	Symbol or Abbreviation	Typical Value	Range of Common Values
Frequency	f	3.5 MHz	2–10 MHz
Period	T	0.3 μs	0.1–0.5 μs
Wavelength	λ	0.4 mm	0.1–0.8 mm
Propagation speed	c	1.54 mm/μs	1.4–1.7 mm/μs
Impedance	z	1,630,000 rayls	1,300,000–1,700,000 rayls
Pulse repetition frequency	PRF	1 kHz	1–10 kHz
Pulse repetition period	PRP	1 ms	0.1–1 ms
Cycles per pulse	n	3	1–5
Pulse duration	PD	1 μs	0.5–3 μs
Spatial pulse length	SPL	1 mm	0.1–1 mm
Duty factor	DF	0.001	0.001–0.01
Spatial peak temporal average intensity	I_{SPTA}	1 mW/cm^2	0.01–100 mW/cm^2
Spatial peak pulse average intensity	I_{SPPA}	1 W/cm^2	0.01–100 W/cm^2
Attenuation coefficient	a_c	3 dB/cm	1–5 dB/cm
Half-intensity depth	HID	1 cm	0.3–1 cm

Table 2.8
Dependence of Various Factors
on Increasing Frequency (↑)

Period ↓
Wavelength ↓
Pulse duration ↓
Duty factor ↓
Spatial pulse length ↓
Attenuation ↑
Half-intensity depth ↓

there may be a reflection when the impedances are equal (if the propagation speeds are different), and there may not be a reflection even if the impedances are different. Scattering occurs at rough media boundaries and within heterogeneous media. The range equation is used to determine distance to reflectors.

Definitions of terms discussed in this chapter are listed below:

Absorption. Conversion of sound to heat.

Acoustic. Having to do with sound.

Acoustic propagation properties. Characteristics of a medium that affect the propagation of sound through it.

Acoustic variables. Pressure, density, temperature, and particle motion—things that vary with space and time in a sound wave.

Amplitude. Maximum variation of an acoustic variable or voltage.

Attenuation. Decrease in amplitude and intensity as a wave travels through a medium.

Attenuation coefficient. Attenuation per unit length of wave travel.

Backscatter. Sound scattered back in the direction from which it originally came.

Beam uniformity ratio. Ratio of the spatial peak to spatial average intensity.

Continuous wave. A wave in which cycles repeat indefinitely, not pulsed.

Continuous-wave mode. Mode of operation in which continuous-wave sound is used.

Coupling medium. Oil or gel used to provide a good sound path between the transducer and the skin.

cw. Abbreviation for continuous wave.

Cycle. Complete variation of an acoustic variable.

dB. Abbreviation for decibel.

Decibel. Unit of power or intensity ratio; the number of decibels is 10 times the logarithm (to the base 10) of the power or intensity ratio.

Density. Mass divided by volume.

Duty factor. Fraction of time that pulsed ultrasound is actually on.

Echo. Reflection.

Effective reflecting area. The area of a reflector from which sound is received by a transducer.

Energy. Capability of doing work.

Frequency. Number of cycles per unit time.

Half-intensity depth. Depth in tissue at which intensity is reduced to one half of what it was at the surface.

Hertz. Unit of frequency, one cycle per second; unit of pulse repetition frequency, one pulse per second.

Impedance. Density multiplied by sound propagation speed.

Incidence angle. Angle between incident sound direction and line perpendicular to boundary of the medium.

Intensity. Power divided by area.

Intensity reflection coefficient. Reflected intensity divided by incident intensity.

Intensity transmission coefficient. Transmitted intensity divided by incident intensity.

Longitudinal wave. Wave in which the particle motion is parallel to the direction of wave travel (compressional wave).

Medium. Material through which a wave travels.

Oblique incidence. Sound direction is not perpendicular to media boundaries.

Particle. Small portion of a medium.

Period. Time per cycle.

Perpendicular. Geometrically related by 90 degrees.

Perpendicular incidence. Sound direction is perpendicular to media boundary.

Propagation. Progression or travel.

Propagation speed. Speed with which a wave moves through a medium.

Pulse. A brief excursion of a quantity from its normal value; a few cycles.

Pulse duration. Time from beginning to end of a pulse.

Pulse repetition frequency. Number of pulses per unit time. Sometimes called pulse repetition rate.

Pulse repetition period. Time from the beginning of a one pulse to the beginning of the next.

Pulsed ultrasound. Ultrasound produced in pulse form by applying electric pulses to the transducer.

Range equation. Relationship between round-trip pulse travel time and distance to a reflector.

Rayl. Unit of impedance; equal to kilogram/meter^2-second.

Reflection. Portion of sound returned from a boundary of a medium.

Reflection angle. Angle between reflected sound direction and line perpendicular to boundary of a medium.

Reflector. Medium boundary that produces a reflection; reflecting surface.

Refraction. Change of sound direction on passing from one medium to another.

Scatterer. An object that scatters sound because of its small size or its surface roughness.

Scattering. Diffusion or redirection of sound in several directions on encountering a particle suspension or a rough surface.

Sound. Traveling wave of acoustic variables.

Spatial pulse length. Length of space over which a pulse occurs.

Specular reflection. Reflection from a smooth boundary.

Transmission angle. Angle between transmitted sound direction and line perpendicular to boundary of a medium.

Ultrasound. Sound of frequency greater than 20 kHz.

Wave. Traveling variation of variables.

Wavelength. Length of space over which a cycle occurs.

Wave variables. Things that are functions of space and time in a wave.

Exercises

2.6.1 Which of the following is a characteristic of a medium through which sound is propagating?
   a. impedance
   b. intensity
   c. amplitude
   d. frequency
   e. period

2.6.2 Which of the following applies to continuous-wave sound?
   a. pulse duration
   b. pulse repetition frequency
   c. frequency
   d. beam uniformity ratio
   e. c and d

2.6.3 Match the following:
   a. frequency: _____   1. time per cycle
   b. period: _____   2. maximum variation per cycle
   c. wavelength: _____   3. length per cycle
   d. propagation speed: _____   4. cycles per second
   e. amplitude: _____   5. speed of a wave through
                                       a medium

2.6.4 Match the following:

   a. wavelength: _____   1. $\dfrac{\text{SPTA intensity}}{\text{SATA intensity}}$

   b. duty factor: _____   2. $\dfrac{\text{propagation speed}}{\text{frequency}}$

   c. intensity: _____   3. $\dfrac{\text{pulse duration}}{\text{pulse repetition period}}$

d. beam uniformity
ratio: _____

4. $\dfrac{\text{power}}{\text{beam area}}$

2.6.5 Match the following:

a. period: _____

1. density x propagation speed

b. pulse repetition period: _____

2. frequency x wavelength

c. impedance: _____

3. $\dfrac{1}{\text{frequency}}$

d. propagation speed: _____

4. $\dfrac{1}{\text{pulse repetition frequency}}$

e. half-intensity depth: _____

5. $\dfrac{3}{\text{attenuation coefficient}}$

f. pulse duration: _____

6. number of cycles in pulse x wavelength

g. spatial pulse length: _____

7. number of cycles in pulse x period

2.6.6 Match the following quantities with their units (answers may be used more than once):

a. frequency: _____   1. s
b. wavelength: _____   2. mm/μs
c. period: _____   3. Hz
d. propagation speed: _____   4. mm
e. pulse duration: _____   5. W/cm^2
f. pulse repetition   6. W
   frequency: _____   7. dB/cm
g. pulse repetition period: _____   8. dB
h. intensity: _____   9. cm^2
i. attenuation: _____
j. attenuation coefficient: _____
k. power: _____
l. beam area: _____
m. half-intensity depth: _____

2.6.7 Match the following (each answer should be used twice):

a. attenuation coefficient = 0.5 dB/cm at 1 MHz: _____   1. soft tissues
b. high attenuation: _____, _____   2. lung
c. high propagation speed: _____   3. bone
d. propagation speed 1.54 mm/μs: _____
e. low propagation speed: _____

2.6.8 Given the following:

> frequency = 2 MHz
> pulse repetition frequency = 1 kHz
> 4 cycles per pulse
> SATA intensity = 1 mW/cm^2
> beam uniformity ratio = 4
> density = 1058 kg/m^3

Applying these values to a soft tissue surface, find the following:

a. propagation speed: _____ mm/µs
b. wavelength: _____ mm
c. spatial pulse length: _____ mm
d. period: _____ µs
e. pulse duration: _____ µs
f. pulse repetition period: _____ ms
g. duty factor: _____
h. SPPA intensity at the surface: _____ W/cm^2
i. attenuation coefficient: _____ dB/cm
j. half-intensity depth: _____ cm
k. attenuation from surface to 3 cm depth: _____ dB
l. intensity ratio corresponding to dB in **k**: _____
m. SATA intensity at 3 cm depth: _____ mW/cm^2
n. SPTA intensity at 3 cm depth: _____ mW/cm^2
o. SAPA intensity at 3 cm depth: _____ mW/cm^2
p. SPPA intensity at 3 cm depth: _____ mW/cm^2
q. impedance: _____ rayls

2.6.9 Which of the following cannot be determined from the others?

a. frequency
b. period
c. amplitude
d. wavelength
e. propagation speed

2.6.10 Which of the following cannot be determined from the others?

a. frequency
b. amplitude
c. intensity
d. power
e. beam area

2.6.11 If density and stiffness are increased, impedance is _____.

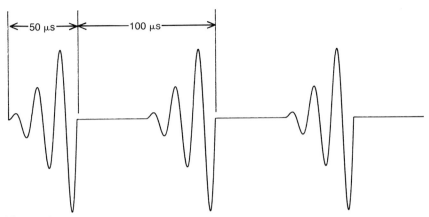

Figure 2.27.

2.6.12 In Figure 2.27, give the pulse repetition period, pulse duration, duty factor, pulse repetition frequency, period, and frequency.

2.6.13 If no refraction occurs as an oblique sound beam passes through the boundary between two materials, the _____ _____ of the materials are known to be _____.

2.6.14 What must be known in order to calculate distance to a reflector?
    a. attenuation, speed, density
    b. attenuation, impedance
    c. attenuation, absorption
    d. travel time, speed
    e. density, speed

2.6.15 With perpendicular incidence, if the impedances of two media are the same, there will be no
    a. inflation
    b. reflection
    c. refraction
    d. calibration
    e. both b and c

2.6.16 What is the transmitted intensity if the incident intensity is 1 mW/cm^2 and the impedances are 1.00 and 2.64 units?
    a. 0.2
    b. 0.4
    c. 0.6
    d. 0.8
    e. 1.0

2.6.17 If the incident intensity is 1 mW/cm^2 and the impedances are 3 and 2 units, the reflected intensity is _____.

2.6.18 No reflection will occur with perpendicular incidence if the media _____ are equal.

2.6.19 No reflection will occur with oblique incidence if the media _____ are equal and the media _____ _____ are equal.

2.6.20 If the incidence angle is 20 degrees and the propagation speeds of media one and two are 1.7 and 1.5 mm/μs, respectively, the transmission angle is _____ degrees.

2.6.21 If the incidence angle is 20 degrees and propagation speeds of media one and two are 1.5 and 1.7 mm/μs, respectively, the transmission angle is _____ degrees.

2.6.22 Scattering occurs at smooth boundaries and within homogeneous media. True or false?

2.6.23 A 3-MHz instrument with an SPTA output intensity of 10 mW/cm^2 images to a maximum depth of 15 cm. In order to image to 18 cm the output intensity of the instrument must be increased to _____ mW/cm^2.

Chapter 3

Transducers

3.1
Introduction

In this chapter we consider the following questions: What is a transducer? How does a transducer generate ultrasound pulses? How does a transducer receive echoes? How are sound beams described and on what do they depend? How are sound beams automatically scanned through tissue cross sections? How is detail resolution described and on what does it depend? The following terms are discussed in this chapter:

annular array	linear phased array
array	linear switched array
axial	matching layer
axial resolution	near zone
bandwidth	operating frequency
continuous mode	piezoelectricity
damping	probe
disc	pulsed mode
electric voltage	quality factor
far zone	resonance frequency
focal length	sensitivity
focal region	side lobes
focus	sound beam
fractional bandwidth	transducer
grating lobes	transducer array
internal focus	transducer assembly
lateral	transducer element
lateral resolution	ultrasound transducer
linear array	voltage pulse

Table 3.1
Transducer Examples

Transducer	converts	to
Light bulb	electricity	light and heat
Automobile engine	chemical energy	motion and heat
Ear	sound	nerve impulses
Oven	electricity	heat
Motor	electricity	motion
Generator	motion	electricity
Battery	chemical energy	electricity
Human body	chemical energy	heat, motion, and sound
Microphone	audible sound	electricity
Loudspeaker	electricity	audible sound

The characteristics of ultrasound that are important for diagnosis have been described in Chapter 2. In this chapter the devices that generate and receive ultrasound are described. They form the connecting link between the ultrasound-tissue interactions of Chapter 2 and the instruments described in Chapters 4 and 6. Except for mention of sound beams in Sections 2.4 and 2.5, the confining of sound to beams has not yet been covered. The devices described in this chapter do not produce sound that travels uniformly in all directions away from the source. Rather, the sound is confined in beams, which are described in Section 3.3.

3.2
Transducers

⑯ Transducers convert one form of energy (Appendix D) to another.* Examples are given in Table 3.1. Ultrasound transducers have no special name, such as a microphone or loudspeaker, which are the names applied to devices that accomplish similar functions with audible sound. Ultrasound transducers convert electric energy into ultrasound energy ⑯ and vice versa. Electric voltages applied to them are converted to ultrasound. Ultrasound incident on them produces electric voltages.

Ultrasound transducers operate on the piezoelectricity (from Greek, πιεζω: to press; ηλεκτρον: amber; amber is an organic resin used in early electrical studies) principle, which was discovered in 1880. The principle

---

* The most general definition of a transducer is a device through which energy can flow from one medium or system to another. The energy conducted by these media or systems may be of the same or different forms. The latter case conforms to the transducer definition given above.

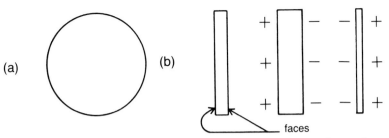

faces

Figure 3.1. A disc transducer element. (a) Front view. (b) Side view with no voltage applied to faces (normal thickness), voltage applied (increased thickness), and voltage of opposite polarity applied (decreased thickness).

states that some materials (ceramics, quartz, and others) produce a voltage when deformed by an applied pressure. Piezoelectricity also results in a production of a pressure when these materials are deformed by an applied voltage. Various formulations of lead zirconate titanate (PZT) are commonly used as materials for production of modern transducer elements. Ceramics such as these are not *naturally* piezoelectric (as quartz is). They are made piezoelectric during production by placing them in a strong electric field while they are at a high temperature.

Single-element transducers (other types are discussed in Section 3.4) are in the form of discs (Fig. 3.1). When an electric voltage is applied to the faces, the thickness of the disc increases or decreases, depending on the polarity of the voltage. The term transducer element (also called piezoelectric element or active element) refers to the piece of piezoelectric material that converts electricity to ultrasound and vice versa. The element with its associated case and damping and matching materials (discussed later in this section) is called the transducer assembly or probe (Fig. 3.2). Both the transducer element and the transducer assembly are commonly referred to as the transducer. Typical diagnostic ultrasound elements are 6 to 19 mm in diameter and 0.2 to 2 mm thick.

Source transducers operated in the continuous mode (continuous-wave mode) are driven by a continuous alternating voltage (see Chapter 6)

Figure 3.2. A transducer assembly or probe. The damping material reduces pulse duration, thus improving axial resolution. The matching layer increases sound transmission into the tissues. The filler material enables the face of the transducer assembly to be flat. The transducer element is usually curved for focusing (see Section 3.3), but it is sometimes flat (unfocused).

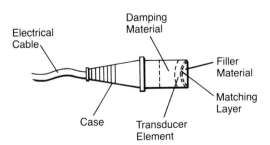

Electrical Cable
Damping Material
Filler Material
Matching Layer
Case
Transducer Element

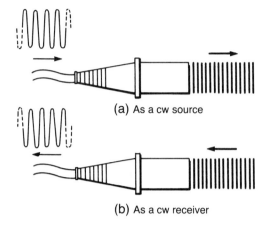

(a) As a cw source

(b) As a cw receiver

Figure 3.3. A transducer assembly operating in the continuous-wave (cw) mode. The device converts (a) a continuous-wave voltage into continuous-wave ultrasound or converts (b) received continuous-wave ultrasound into a continuous-wave voltage.

and produce an alternating pressure that propagates as a sound wave (Fig. 3.3[a]). The frequency of the sound produced is equal to the frequency of the driving voltage. The operating frequency (sometimes called resonance frequency) of the transducer is its preferred frequency of operation. Operating frequency is determined by the propagation speed of the transducer material (typically 4 to 6 mm/μs) and the thickness (Table 3.2) of the transducer element.

$$\text{operating frequency (MHz)} = \frac{\text{propagation speed (mm/μs)}}{2 \times \text{thickness (mm)}} \qquad f_o = \frac{c_m}{2w}$$

where propagation speed is that for the transducer material

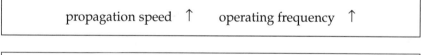

propagation speed ↑   operating frequency ↑

thickness ↑   operating frequency ↓

Continuous-wave sound encountering a receiving transducer is converted to a continuous alternating voltage (Fig. 3.3[b]). For instruments employing the continuous-wave mode, separate source and receiver transducer elements are required, as they each must continuously perform their function. These elements are built into a single transducer assembly.

Table 3.2
Transducer Element Thickness*
for Various Frequencies

Frequency (MHz)	Thickness (mm)
2.0	1.0
3.5	0.6
5.0	0.4
7.5	0.3
10.0	0.2

*Assuming element propagation speed
of 4 mm/μs.

Source transducers operated in the pulsed mode (pulsed ultrasound) are driven by voltage pulses (see Section 4.2) and produce ultrasound pulses (Fig. 3.4). These transducers convert received reflections into voltage pulses. The pulse repetition frequency is equal to the voltage pulse repetition frequency, which is determined by the instrument driving the transducer. The pulse duration is equal to the period (one over operating frequency) multiplied by the number of cycles in the pulse (see Section 2.3). Damping material (a mixture of metal powder and a plastic or epoxy) is attached to the rear face of the transducer element to reduce the number of cycles in each pulse (Fig. 3.5). This reduces pulse duration and spatial pulse length and thus results in improved axial resolution (Section 3.5). This method of damping is analogous to packing foam rubber around a bell that is rung by a tap with a hammer. The rubber reduces the time that the bell rings following the tap. It also reduces the loudness or intensity of the ringing.

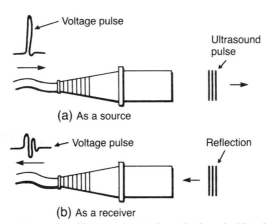

(a) As a source

(b) As a receiver

Figure 3.4. A transducer assembly operating in the pulsed mode. This device converts (a) electric voltage pulses into ultrasound pulses and converts (b) received ultrasound pulses (reflections) into electric voltage pulses.

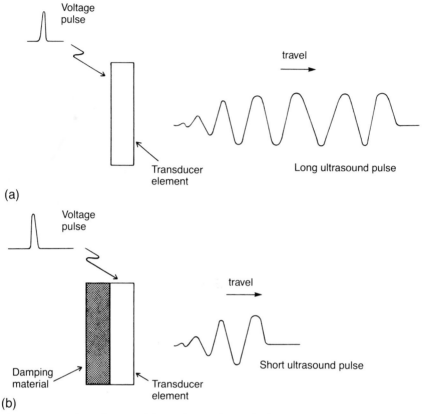

Figure 3.5. Without damping (a), a voltage pulse applied to transducer element results in a long pulse of many cycles. With damping material on the rear face of the transducer element (b), application of a voltage pulse results in a short pulse of a few cycles. This figure shows each pulse traveling away from the transducer from left to right in space so that the right-hand end is the beginning or leading edge of the pulse.

For ultrasound transducers, the damping material reduces the ultrasound amplitude and thus decreases the efficiency and sensitivity of the system (undesired effect). This is the price paid for reduced spatial pulse length (desired effect resulting in improved axial resolution). Some damping may also be accomplished electrically within the instrument. Typically, pulses of two or three cycles are generated with diagnostic ultrasound transducers.

A matching layer is commonly placed on the transducer face (Fig. 3.2). This material has an impedance intermediate between those of the transducer element and the tissue. It reduces the reflection of ultrasound at the transducer element surface, improving sound transmission across it. This is analogous to the coating layer on a camera lens, which reduces light reflection at the air-glass boundary. The optimum thickness for this matching layer is one quarter of a wavelength. Because many frequencies and wavelengths are present in short ultrasound pulses (see later this section), multiple matching layers provide a greater improvement in sound transmission across the element-tissue boundary.

Because of its very low impedance, even a very thin layer of air between the transducer and the skin surface will reflect virtually all the sound, preventing any penetration into the tissue. For this reason, a coupling medium, usually an aqueous gel or mineral oil, is applied to the skin before transducer contact. This eliminates the air layer and permits the sound to pass into the tissue.

A transducer operating in the pulsed mode preferentially produces a frequency equal to its operating frequency (introduced earlier in this section). However, the ultrasound pulses produced contain frequencies in addition to this. The shorter the pulse (the fewer the number of cycles), the more frequencies that are present. The range of frequencies involved in a pulse is called its bandwidth (Fig. 3.6). Bandwidth must be specified by some definition of where in the frequency range to stop. For example, a 6-dB bandwidth is the range of frequencies including those that have half or greater the amplitude of the strongest one (operating frequency). Fractional bandwidth is equal to the bandwidth divided by the operating frequency. Quality factor (Q factor) is equal to operating frequency divided by the bandwidth, that is, one divided by the fractional bandwidth.

$$\text{quality factor} = \frac{\text{operating frequency (MHz)}}{\text{bandwidth (MHz)}} \qquad Q = \frac{f_o}{BW}$$

operating frequency ↑	quality factor ↑

bandwidth ↑	quality factor ↓

Quality factor is unitless. The inclusion of damping material in the transducer assembly increases the bandwidth and decreases the quality factor. For short (two or three cycle) pulses, the quality factor is approximately equal to the number of cycles in the pulse. The overall

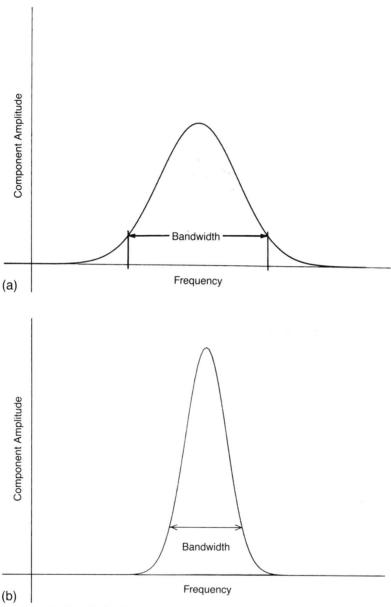

Figure 3.6. A plot of the frequencies present in an ultrasound pulse. Component amplitude is the amplitude of each frequency component present. Bandwidth is the frequency range within which the amplitudes exceed some reference value. Plot (a) represents a broad band, low quality factor, damped pulse. Plot (b) represents a narrow band, high quality factor, undamped pulse.

system bandwidth is determined not only by the transducer but also by the instrument electronics.

Exercises

3.2.1 A transducer converts one form of _____ to another.

3.2.2 Ultrasound transducers convert _____ energy into _____ energy and vice versa.

3.2.3 Ultrasound transducers operate on the _____ principle.

3.2.4 Single-element transducers are in the form of _____.

3.2.5 The _____ of a transducer element changes when a voltage is applied to the faces.

3.2.6 The term transducer is often used to refer to either a transducer _____ or a transducer _____.

3.2.7 A transducer _____ is part of a transducer _____.

3.2.8 A continuously alternating voltage applied to a transducer produces _____ ultrasound.

3.2.9 Electric voltage pulses applied to a transducer produce ultrasound _____.

3.2.10 Operating frequency _____ as transducer element thickness is increased.

3.2.11 Addition of damping material to a transducer reduces the number of _____ in the pulse, thus improving _____ _____. It increases the _____ and decreases the _____ _____.

3.2.12 Addition of damping material reduces the _____ and _____ of the diagnostic system.

3.2.13 Ultrasound transducers typically generate pulses of _____ or _____ cycles.

3.2.14 If the propagation speed of the transducer element material is 4 mm/μs, the thickness required for an operating frequency of 10 MHz is _____ mm.

3.2.15 If the propagation speed of the transducer element material is 6 mm/μs, the operating frequency for a thickness of 0.2 mm is _____ MHz.

3.2.16 The matching layer on the transducer surface reduces _____ caused by impedance difference.

3.2.17 A coupling medium on the skin surface eliminates reflection caused by _____.

3.2.18 Quality factor is given in
    a. MHz
    b. mm/μs
    c. per cent
    d. all of the above
    e. none of the above
3.2.19 Increasing the bandwidth increases the quality factor. True or false?
3.2.20 The range of _____ involved in an ultrasound pulse is called its bandwidth.
3.2.21 A two-cycle pulse has a Q factor of approximately _____.
    a. 0.2
    b. 0.5
    c. 2
    d. 5
    e. 20
3.2.22 If bandwidth is 1 MHz and operating frequency is 3 MHz, calculate the following:
    a. Q factor _____
    b. fractional bandwidth _____
    c. lowest frequency _____
    d. highest frequency _____
    e. approximate number of cycles per pulse _____

3.3
Beams and Focusing

The ultrasound pulse generated by the (flat) disc transducer in Figure 3.1 is contained in a cylindrical shape, as shown in Figure 3.7. The spatial pulse length was discussed in Sections 2.3 and 3.2. This section is concerned with the pulse diameter. The sound beam is a description of this diameter as the pulse travels away from the transducer.

A single-element (flat) disc transducer operating in the continuous-wave mode produces a sound beam with a beam diameter that varies according to the distance from the transducer face, as shown in Figure 3.8. The intensity is not uniform throughout the beam (Section 2.4). The beam diameter shown in Figure 3.8 approximates that portion of the sound produced that is greater than 4 per cent of the spatial peak intensity. This particular value was chosen because it gives the simplest picture.

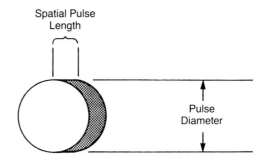

Figure 3.7. An ultrasound pulse generated by a single-element disc transducer driven by an electrical voltage pulse as shown in Figure 3.4. The pulse diameter is equal to beam diameter. This varies with distance from the transducer (Fig. 3.8). Spatial pulse length is described in Figure 2.9.

The 6-dB beam diameter that is often used is narrower than that pictured in Figure 3.8. It includes that portion of the sound that is greater than 25 percent of the spatial peak intensity. Sometimes significant intensity travels out in some directions not included in the beam as pictured. These additional "beams" are called side lobes. They are really "cone" or "ring" beams for a disc transducer.

The region from the disc out to a distance of one near-zone length is called the near zone, near field, or Fresnel zone. Near-zone length (also called near-field length) is given by the following equations:

$$\text{near-zone length (mm)} = \frac{[\text{transducer diameter (mm)}]^2}{4 \times \text{wavelength (mm)}} \qquad NZL = \frac{D_T^2}{4\lambda}$$

For soft tissues:

$$\text{near-zone length (mm)} \overset{*}{=} \frac{[\text{transducer diameter (mm)}]^2 \times \text{frequency (MHz)}}{6} \qquad NZL \times \frac{D_T^2 f}{6}$$

diameter ↑   near-zone length ↑

frequency ↑   near-zone length ↑

The second equation is derived from the first by substituting, for wavelength, propagation speed (1.54 mm/μs for soft tissues) divided by frequency. Table 3.3 lists near-zone lengths for various transducer frequencies and diameters.

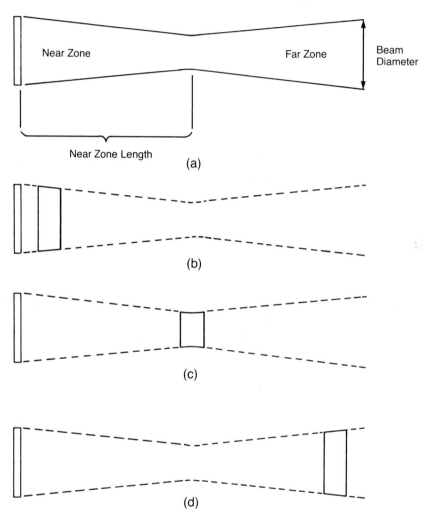

Figure 3.8. Beam diameter for a single-element unfocused disc transducer operating in the continuous wave mode (a). This diameter approximates the region of that portion of the sound produced that is greater than 4 per cent of the spatial peak intensity. The near zone is the region between the disc and the minimum beam diameter. The far zone is the region beyond the minimum beam diameter. Intensity is not constant within the beam, with intensity variations being greatest in the near zone. The beam diameter in (a) approximates the changing pulse diameter as an ultrasound pulse travels away from the transducer. (b) A pulse shortly after leaving the transducer. (c) Later the pulse is located at the end of the near-zone length, where its diameter is a minimum. (d) Still later the pulse is in the far zone, where its diameter is increasing as it travels. This figure assumes a nonscattering, nonrefracting medium such as water.

Table 3.3
Near-zone Length (NZL) for
Unfocused Transducers

Frequency (MHz)	Diameter (mm)	NZL (cm)
2.25	19	13
3.5	13	10
3.5	19	20
5.0	6	3
5.0	10	8
5.0	13	14
7.5	6	4
10.0	6	6

The region beyond a distance of one near-zone length is called the far zone, far field, or Fraunhofer zone.

The beam diameter depends on

1. wavelength (therefore frequency)
2. transducer diameter
3. distance from transducer

In the approximation of Figure 3.8, at a distance of one near-zone length from the transducer, the beam diameter is equal to one half the transducer diameter. At a distance of two times the near-zone length, the beam diameter is equal to the transducer diameter. Beyond this distance, the beam diameter increases in proportion to distance.

The diameter of an ultrasound pulse (Fig. 3.7) is equal to the beam diameter (Fig. 3.8) for the distance from the transducer face at which the pulse is located at any given time. As the pulse travels through the near zone, its diameter decreases; as it travels through the far zone, its diameter increases.

A beam description different than that of Figure 3.8 is often seen (Fig. 3.9). Beam characteristics in the near zone are complicated. It is desirable to provide a simplified, although approximate, picture of this behavior. Figure 3.9 is one such approach. However, a more accurate description is given in Figure 3.8, which indicates that the beam narrows to a minimum diameter at approximately the location of the transition from the near to the far zone.

It is important to realize that even for flat, unfocused transducer elements (Figs. 3.8 and 3.9), there is some beam narrowing or "focusing." The beam diameter approximates the changing pulse diameter as an ultrasound pulse travels away from the transducer. With the 4 per cent beam of Figure 3.8, this diameter reduces to approximately one half of the transducer element diameter at the transition from near to far zone. The diameter then increases in the far zone.

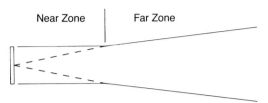

Figure 3.9. Traditional presentation of the beam for a flat disc transducer element. A more accurate view, using a 4 per cent intensity beam diameter, is given in Figure 3.8.

Sound beams produced by disc transducers have beam areas given by the following equation:

$$\text{beam area (cm}^2) = 0.8 \times [\text{beam diameter (cm)}^2] \qquad A_B = 0.8\, D_B^2$$

$$\text{beam diameter } \uparrow \qquad \text{beam area } \uparrow$$

Example 3.3.1

For soft tissue and a 10-mm 5-MHz transducer, what are the beam diameters 8 and 16 cm from the transducer? First find the near-zone length:

$$\text{near-zone length} = \frac{(\text{transducer diameter})^2 \times \text{frequency}}{6}$$

$$\frac{10^2 \times 5}{6} = 83 \text{ mm} = 8.3 \text{ cm}$$

A distance of 8 cm is therefore near the end of the near zone. The beam diameter is therefore approximately equal to one half the transducer element diameter, i.e., 5 mm. A distance of 16 cm is in the far zone at approximately double the near-zone length. Therefore, the beam diameter at this point is approximately equal to the transducer element diameter, 10 mm.

The effects of frequency on near-zone length are shown in Figure 3.10. The effects of transducer diameter are shown in Figure 3.11. The beam dimensions for those figures are calculated in Exercises 3.3.11 through 3.3.18.

An increase in frequency or transducer size increases the near-zone length. When sufficiently far from the transducer, increasing frequency

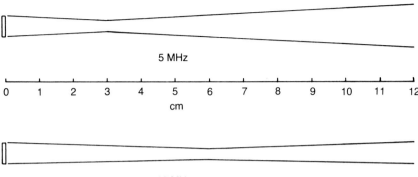

Figure 3.10. Beams for 6-mm diameter disc transducers of two frequencies. Higher frequency produces smaller beam diameter (beyond 4 cm) and longer near-zone length.

or the transducer size can decrease the beam diameter (Figs. 3.10 and 3.11).

The beam in Figure 3.8(a) is for continuous-wave mode and is used to describe pulses in the rest of the figure. The beam for pulses is not exactly the same as for continuous sound. One important reason for this is that the beam is a result of Huygens' principle, which states that each small portion of the surface of a transducer may be considered as a separate (omnidirectional) source. The beam is a result of combining the resulting sound emanating from all the small sources. For short pulses, this combination process is altered. Another reason why pulse beams are different is because pulses contain many frequencies. Because a beam depends on frequency, many beams are produced for a wide-bandwidth pulse. The combination of all of these results in the actual pulse beam

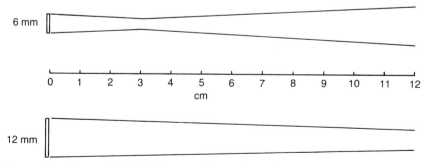

Figure 3.11. Beams for 5-MHz disc transducers of two diameters. The larger transducer produces the larger near-zone length. The right-hand portion of the figure shows that a smaller transducer can produce a larger-diameter beam. The beam diameters are equal at a distance of 8 cm.

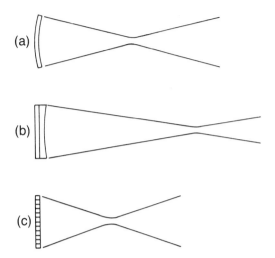

Figure 3.12. Sound focusing by (a) a curved transducer, (b) a lens, and (c) a phased array. Lenses focus because the propagation speed through them is higher than that through tissues. Refraction (see Section 2.5) at the surface of the lens forms the beam such that a focal region occurs. The operation of phased arrays is described in Section 3.4. The amount by which the beam diameter is reduced by focusing is described qualitatively as weak or strong focus.

produced. As lateral resolution depends on beam diameter, which depends on pulse duration, axial and lateral resolutions are not independent.

For improved lateral resolution (Section 3.5), beam diameter is reduced by focusing the sound in a manner similar to the focusing of light. Sound may be focused (Fig. 3.12) by employing a curved (rather than a flat) transducer element, a curved reflector in the transducer assembly, a lens, or a phased array (see Section 3.4). "Internal focus" refers to the use of a curved transducer element. Beam diameter is decreased in the focal region and between it and the transducer; it is widened in the region beyond (Fig. 3.13). Focal length is the distance from the transducer to the center of the focal region or to the location of the spatial peak intensity. Manufacturers use qualitative terms such as short, medium, or long internal focus to indicate the length of focal regions or focal length. The two normally go together, i.e., long focal lengths are associated with long focal regions. Numerical values associated with these terms vary with manufacturers. The focal length cannot be greater than the near-zone length of the comparable (same transducer diameter and operating frequency) unfocused transducers. Focal zone is specified as the distance between two points at the center of the beam at which the intensity is some fraction (commonly 25 per cent, 6 dB) of the peak intensity at the focus. A second way of specifying focal zone is the distance between equal beam widths or diameters that are some multiple (e.g., two times) of the minimum value (at the focus). Most diagnostic transducers are focused to some degree.

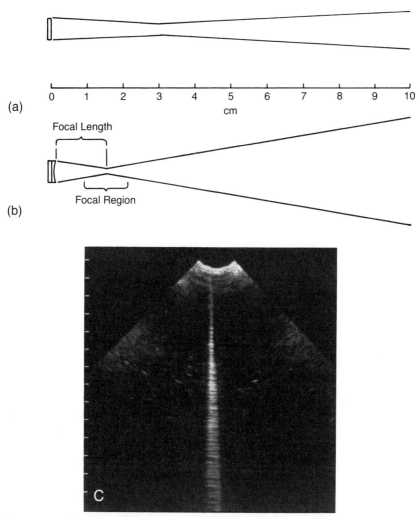

Figure 3.13. Beam diameter for 6-mm 5-MHz disc transducer of Figure 3.9 and 3.10 without (a) and with (b) a focusing lens. Focusing in this case produces a minimum beam diameter that is half that produced without focusing. However, beyond 2.5 cm from the transducer (outside the focal region), the focused beam diameter is greater than the unfocused. (c) A focused beam from a 5-MHz, 19-mm diameter transducer. This is an ultrasound image of a beam profile test object (Chapter 7), which contains a thin vertical scattering layer down the center. Scanning this object generates a picture of the beam profile (the pulse width at all depths). In this case the focus occurs at about 4 cm depth (this image has a total depth of 15 cm).

Exercises

3.3.1 The beam diameter in Figure 3.8 includes that portion of the sound produced that is greater than _____ per cent of the spatial peak intensity.

3.3.2 The beam is divided into two regions called the _____ zone and the _____ zone.

3.3.3 The dividing point between the two regions is at a distance from the transducer equal to one _____ length.

3.3.4 Beam diameter depends on _____, transducer _____, and _____ from the transducer.

3.3.5 Near-zone length is proportional to the square of the _____ and inversely proportional to _____.

3.3.6 For a given medium (a given propagation speed), near-zone length is proportional to the square of the _____ _____ and to the _____.

3.3.7 At a distance of one near-zone length from the transducer, beam diameter is equal to _____ transducer diameter.

3.3.8 At a distance of _____ times the near-zone length, beam diameter is equal to transducer diameter.

3.3.9 In the near zone, beam diameter _____ as distance from the transducer increases.

3.3.10 In the far zone, beam diameter _____ as distance from the transducer increases.

3.3.11 For soft tissue and a 6-mm 5-MHz transducer (Figs. 3.10 and 3.11), the near-zone length is _____ mm.

3.3.12 For Exercise 3.3.11, the beam diameters at distances of 15, 30, 60, and 120 mm from the transducer are _____, _____, _____, and _____ mm, respectively.

3.3.13 For soft tissue and a 6-mm 10-MHz transducer (Fig. 3.10), the near-zone length is _____ mm.

3.3.14 For Exercise 3.3.13, the beam diameters at 60, 120, and 180 mm from the transducer are _____, _____, and _____ mm, respectively.

3.3.15 In Exercises 3.3.11 to 3.3.14, the higher-frequency transducer produces the _____ near-zone length and the _____ beam diameter at 60 mm from the transducer.

3.3.16 For soft tissue and a 12-mm 5-MHz transducer (Fig. 3.11), the near-zone length is _____ mm.

3.3.17 For Exercise 3.3.16, the beam diameters at 60, 120, 180, and 240 mm from the transducer are _____, _____, _____, and _____ mm, respectively.

3.3.18 In Exercises 3.3.11, 3.3.12, 3.3.16, and 3.3.17, the larger transducer

produces   the   _____   near-zone   length   and   the
_____ beam diameter at 120 mm from the transducer.

3.3.19 Doubling the transducer diameter _____ the near-zone
length.

3.3.20 Doubling the frequency _____ the near-zone length.

3.3.21 If transducer diameter is doubled and frequency is halved, the
near-zone length is _____.

3.3.22 Sound may be focused by employing a
   a. curved element
   b. curved reflector
   c. lens
   d. phased array
   e. more than one of the above

3.3.23 Focusing reduces the beam diameter at all distances from the
transducer. True or false?

3.3.24 _____   _____ is the distance from the
transducer to the location of the spatial peak intensity produced
by a focused transducer.

3.4
Automatic Scanning

There are two ways in which automatic scanning of a sound beam
can be performed:

1. mechanical scan
2. electronic scan

Both of these methods provide means for sweeping the sound beam
through the tissues rapidly and repeatedly. The first method may be accomplished by oscillating a transducer in angle, by rotating a transducer
or a group of transducers, by oscillating a reflector, or by linearly
translating a transducer. In most mechanical real-time transducers, the
rotating or oscillating component is immersed in a coupling liquid
within the transducer assembly. The sound beam is thus swept at a rapid
rate without movement of the entire transducer assembly. Approaches to
mechanical scanning are shown in Figure 3.14.

Electronic scanning is performed with arrays. Transducer arrays are
transducer assemblies with several transducer elements. The elements
are rectangular in shape and arranged in a line (linear array) or are ring-
shaped and arranged concentrically (annular array) (Fig. 3.15).

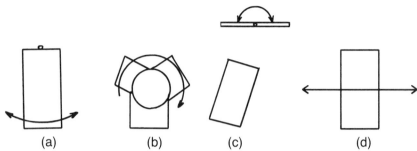

Figure 3.14. Mechanical real-time transducer types. (a) Oscillating transducer; (b) rotating group of transducers; (c) oscillating mirror (stationary transducer); (d) linearly translating transducer.

A linear switched array (sometimes called a linear sequenced array or simply a linear array) is operated by applying voltage pulses to groups of elements in succession (Fig. 3.16). Each group of elements acts like a larger transducer element in this case. The origin of the sound beam moves across the face of the transducer assembly and thus produces the same effect as manual linear scanning with a single-element transducer. Such electronic scanning, however, can be done in a more rapid and more consistent manner. If this electronic scanning is repeated rapidly enough, a real-time (Section 4.5) presentation of information can result. This requires scanning across the transducer assembly several times per second.

A linear phased array (commonly called a phased array) is operated by applying voltage pulses to all elements in the assembly as a complete group, but with small time differences, so that the resulting sound pulse may be shaped and steered (Fig. 3.17). If the same time differences are

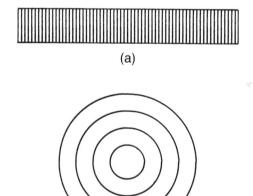

(a)

(b)

Figure 3.15. Front views of (a) a linear array with 64 rectangular elements and (b) an annular array with four elements.

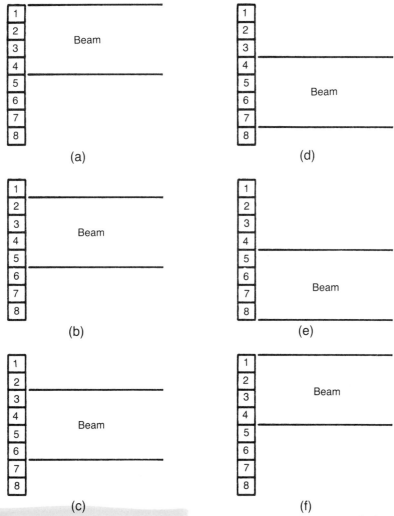

Figure 3.16. A linear switched array (side view). Voltage pulses are applied simultaneously to all elements in a group: first to elements 1 through 4 as a group (a), next to elements 2 through 5 (b), and so on across the transducer assembly (c–e). Then the process is repeated (f).

used each time the process is repeated, the same beam shape and direction will result repeatedly. However, the time differences may be changed with each successive repetition, so that the beam shape (Fig. 3.18) or direction (Fig. 3.19) can continually change. This can then result in sweeping of the beam (the beam direction changes with each pulse) and in variable focusing (the focal length changes with each pulse).

A linear phased array can focus or steer electronically only in the scan plane (the vertical plane in Fig. 3.17). Focus (fixed) can be achieved

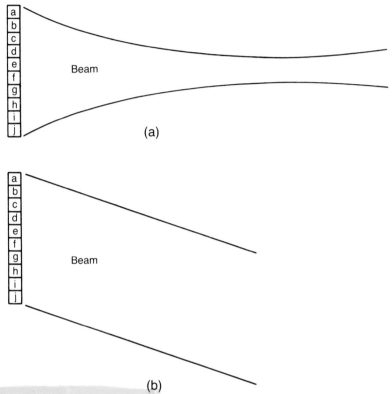

Figure 3.17. A linear phased array (side view). (a) By applying voltage pulses to the upper and lower elements earlier than to the middle elements, the beam can be focused. (b) By applying voltage pulses to the upper elements earlier than to the lower elements, the beam can be steered down. Similarly, by applying voltage pulses to the lower elements earlier, the beam can be steered up. Pulses may be applied in such a way that parts (a) and (b) are combined, resulting in a focused and steered beam.

in the other plane with a lens. A linear array can be operated simultaneously as a switched and phased array, providing scanning, steering, and shaping of the beam. Annular phased arrays (Fig. 3.15[b]) can focus in both planes but cannot provide beam steering. The addition of an oscillating mirror to these arrays provides a means for beam steering.

When an array is receiving reflections, the electrical outputs of the elements can be timed so that the array "listens" in a particular direction with a listening focus at a particular depth. This received focus depth may be continually increased as the transmitted pulse travels through the tissues. This continually changing received focus is called dynamic focusing.

In addition to side lobes, which single-element transducers have (Section 3.3), arrays have grating lobes, which are additional beams resulting from their multielement structure.

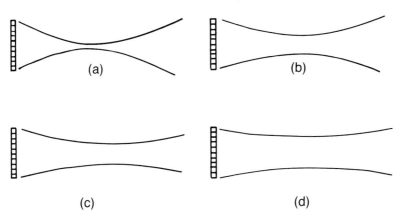

Figure 3.18. Variable focusing with a linear phased array. In the sequence (a) through (d), the time delays between applications of the electrical pulse to the elements are reduced. This results in weakening of the focus and a movement of the focus away from the transducer assembly. In some instruments, the delay can be controlled by the operator so that focal depth can be selected.

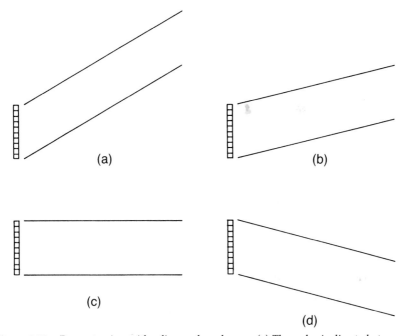

Figure 3.19. Beam steering with a linear phased array. (a) The pulse is directed at an upward angle because the voltage pulse from the instrument pulser is applied to the elements in rapid succession from bottom to top. (b) The next pulse travels out at less of an upward angle because the time delays in applying the voltage pulse to the elements are less than in (a). (c) The next pulse travels out horizontally because the voltage pulse is applied simultaneously to all the elements. (d) The next pulse is directed at a downward angle because the voltage pulse is applied in rapid succession to the elements from top to bottom.

Exercises

3.4.1 Transducer arrays are transducer assemblies with more than one transducer _____.

3.4.2 Two types of arrays are _____ and _____.

3.4.3 Linear arrays are of two types according to how they are operated: linear _____ arrays and linear _____ arrays.

3.4.4 Match the following (answers may be used more than once):

    a. A linear switched array   1. scan
       can _____ the   2. steer
       beam.   3. shape

    b. A linear switched array
       cannot _____ or
       _____ the beam.

    c. A linear phased array can
       _____ and
       _____ the beam.

    d. An annular phased array
       can _____ the beam but
       cannot _____ or
       _____ the beam.

    e. A combined linear
       switched and phased array
       can _____,
       _____, and
       _____ the beam.

3.4.5 A linear array can scan, steer, or shape in _____ dimension(s).

3.4.6 An annular array can shape in _____ dimension(s).

3.4.7 An annular array can steer a beam with the aid of an _____ _____.

3.4.8. Match the following (answers may be used more than once).

    a. linear switched array: 1. Voltage pulses are applied in
       _____   succession to groups of elements.
    b. linear phased array: _____ 2. Voltage pulses are applied to all
    c. annular phased array: elements as a group, but with
       _____   small time differences.

3.4.9. In Figure 3.17, if elements are pulsed in rapid succession in the order a, b, c, d, e, f, g, h, i, j, the resulting beam is

    a. steered up
    b. steered down
    c. focused

3.4.10. In Figure 3.17, if elements are pulsed in rapid succession in the order j, i, h, g, f, e, d, c, b, a, the resulting beam is
  a. steered up
  b. steered down
  c. focused
3.4.11. In Figure 3.17, if elements are pulsed in rapid succession in order a and j, b and i, c and h, d and g, and e and f, the resulting beam is
  a. steered up
  b. steered down
  c. focused

3.5
Resolution

(45) There are two primary aspects to resolution in imaging: detail (geometric) resolution and contrast (gray-scale) resolution. The latter is discussed in Chapter 4 (Section 4.4). If two reflectors are not sufficiently separated, they will not produce separate reflections and thus will not be separated on the instrument display. Characteristics of the instrument electronics and display may further degrade this detail resolution. It is apparent, however, that if separate reflections are not initially generated the reflectors will not be separated on the display. In ultrasound imaging (46) there are two aspects to detail resolution: axial and lateral. They depend on different characteristics of the ultrasound pulses as they travel through the tissues.

The important parameter in determining the required separation for resolution along the direction of the sound travel (axial resolution) is the spatial pulse length (Section 2.3). The axial resolution is the minimum reflector separation required along the direction of sound travel so that separate reflections will be produced (Fig. 3.20). It is also called longitudinal, range, or depth resolution.

$$\text{axial resolution (mm)} = \frac{\text{spatial pulse length (mm)}}{2} \qquad R_A = \frac{SPL}{2}$$

For soft tissues:
$$\text{axial resolution (mm)} \stackrel{*}{=} \frac{0.77 \times \text{number of cycles in the pulse}}{\text{frequency (MHz)}} \qquad R_A \stackrel{*}{=} \frac{0.77n}{f}$$

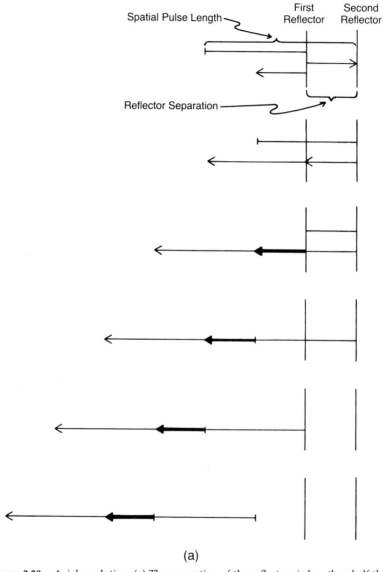

(a)

Figure 3.20. Axial resolution. (a) The separation of the reflectors is less than half the spatial pulse length, so that reflection overlap occurs. Separate reflections are not produced. The reflectors are not resolved.

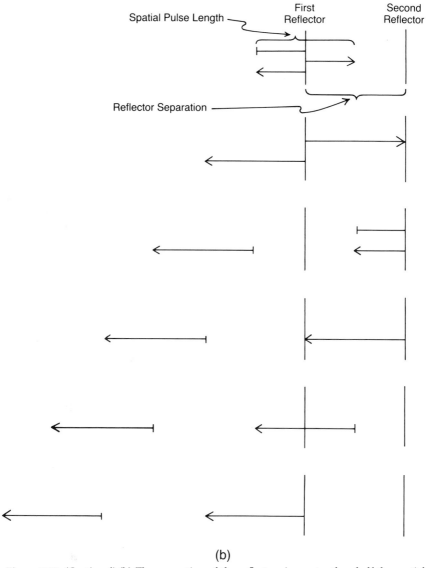

(b)

Figure 3.20. *(Continued)* (b) The separation of the reflectors is greater than half the spatial pulse length, so that reflection overlap does not occur. Separate reflections are produced and the reflectors are resolved. Action proceeds in time from top to bottom in each part of the figure.

spatial pulse length ↑	axial resolution ↑

cycles per pulse ↑	axial resolution ↑

frequency ↑	axial resolution ↓

The second equation is derived from the first by substituting for spatial pulse length according to the last equation in the box on page 24.

 Axial resolution is like a golf score—the smaller the better. The smaller it is, the more detail that can be displayed and the closer two reflectors can be along the sound path and still be seen distinctly. To improve axial resolution, spatial pulse length must be reduced. Because spatial pulse length is the product of wavelength and the number of cycles in the pulse (see Section 2.3), one or both of these must be reduced. For a given propagation speed (such as 1.54 mm/μs in soft tissue), wavelength is reduced as frequency is increased (see Section 2.2). The number of cycles in each pulse may be reduced by increasing transducer damping; this was discussed in Section 3.2. If the number of cycles per pulse is reduced to a minimum (two or three), the only way to further improve axial resolution is to increase frequency:

Axial resolution improves as frequency increases.

When this is done, however, there is a price to be paid. It is a reduction in imaging depth (Section 2.4), because attenuation increases as frequency increases:

Imaging depth decreases as frequency increases.

 In order to reasonably meet resolution and imaging depth requirements, the useful frequency range is restricted to between 2 and 10 MHz. The lower portion of the range is useful when large depth (e.g., an

obese subject) or high attenuation is encountered. The higher portion of
the frequency range is useful when small depth is required (e.g., in imag-
~~ing the breast, eye,~~ thyroid, or superficial vessels or in pediatric imag-
ients, 3.5 MHz is a satisfactory frequency, whereas
hildren, 5 and 7.5 MHz can often be used. If fre-
Hz are used, the axial resolution is not sufficient. If
n 10 MHz (less than 10 MHz in many applications)
not sufficient.

alues for half-intensity depth (from Table 2.5) and
al resolution for various frequencies. Half-intensity
is equal to 60 divided by frequency in megahertz.
illimeters for a two-cycle pulse in soft tissue is equal
requency in megahertz. Therefore, for a two-cycle
half-intensity depth is approximately 40 times axial

on is the minimum separation (in the direction per-
rection of sound travel or the direction of the beam)
ors such that when the beam is scanned across them,
two separate reflections are produced (Fig. 3.21). Lateral resolution is
equal to beam diameter.

---

lateral resolution (mm) = beam diameter (mm) $R_1 = D_B$

Recall that beam diameter varies with distance from the transducer,
and therefore so does lateral resolution. If the lateral separation between
two reflectors is greater than the beam diameter, two separate reflections
are produced when the beam is scanned across them. Thus they are
resolved, i.e., detected as separate reflectors.

Lateral resolution is also called transverse, angular, and azimuthal
resolution. As with axial resolution, a smaller value indicates an improvement (finer detail is imaged). Lateral resolution may be improved
by reducing the beam diameter. This may be done by increasing the frequency. Recall that increasing the frequency also improves axial resolution, but at the expense of decreasing the half-intensity depth. A smaller
transducer improves lateral resolution near the transducer, but makes it
worse farther out (e.g., at 10 cm from the transducer in Figure 3.11). The
primary means for reducing beam diameter and improving lateral
resolution is focusing (Fig. 3.12).

Because ultrasound pulses used in imaging do not have constant
amplitude (Fig. 2.15), the overlapping and separation concept of resolution in this section needs further discussion. How much can the pulses

Table 3.4
Half-intensity Depth and Axial Resolution
(Two-Cycle Pulse) in Tissue

Frequency (MHz)	Half-intensity Depth (mm)	Axial Resolution (mm)
1.00	60	1.5
2.25	27	0.7
3.50	17	0.4
5.00	12	0.3
7.50	8	0.2
10.00	6	0.2

overlap and still be distinguished? This depends on the contrast resolution of the imaging system (Section 4.5). The better it is, the better the detail (axial and lateral) resolution. This is because even with overlap, pulses can have a dip in their combined amplitude (Fig. 3.22). If the contrast resolution of the system can sense this dip, the echoes can be resolved. Thus, contrast resolution and detail resolution interact and are not independent. This also means that detail resolutions are *related to*, not necessarily *equal to*, spatial pulse length and beam diameter.

Diagnostic ultrasound transducers normally have better axial resolution than lateral resolution, although the two may be comparable in the focal region of strongly focused beams. Imaging system resolution is normally not quite as good as transducer (acoustic) resolution discussed in this section. The resolution of the imaging system (ability to display detail) will be no better than the acoustic resolution. It may be slightly worse, because electronics and the display can degrade resolution. Figures 3.23 to 3.25 show examples of typical detail resolutions.

Exercises

3.5.1 Axial resolution is the minimum reflector separation required along the direction of _____ _____ so that separate _____ are produced.
3.5.2 Axial resolution depends directly on _____ _____ _____.
3.5.3 The smaller the axial resolution is, the better it is. True or false?
3.5.4 If there are three cycles of 1-mm wavelength in a pulse, the axial resolution is _____ mm.
3.5.5 For pulses traveling through soft tissue in which frequency is 3 MHz and there are 4 cycles per pulse, the axial resolution is _____ mm.
3.5.6 If there are three cycles per pulse, the axial resolution in soft tissue at the extremes of the useful frequency range for diagnostic ultrasound are _____ and _____ mm.

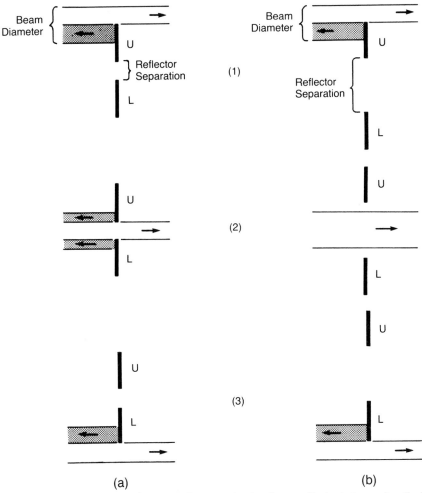

Figure 3.21. Lateral resolution. (a) Reflector separation (perpendicular to beam direction) is less than beam diameter. (b) Reflector separation is greater than beam diameter. (1) Sound travels from left to right and encounters the upper reflector (U), with part of the beam (shaded) being reflected back toward the source and the remainder continuing past the reflector. (2) The beam has been scanned down so that (a) it is partially reflected by both upper and lower (L) reflectors or so that (b) no reflection occurs, the beam passing completely between the reflectors. (3) The beam has been scanned down further so that part of it is reflected by the lower reflector, the remainder continuing past the reflector. (a) The scanning sequence 1-2-3 results in continual reflection from one or both of the reflectors. Separate reflections are not produced, and the reflectors are not resolved. (b) The scanning sequence 1-2-3 results in reflection from the upper reflector, then no reflection, then reflection from the lower reflector. Separate reflections are produced, and the reflectors are resolved.

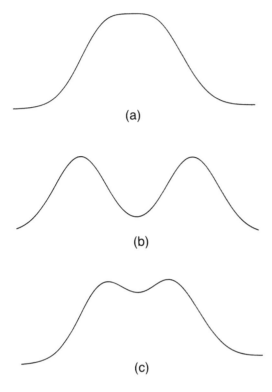

(a)

(b)

(c)

Figure 3.22. (a) Two echo pulses that overlap enough so that there is no amplitude dip between them. These cannot be distinguished by the instrument. Therefore, they will be presented as one and be unresolved. (b) Significantly less overlap (significantly greater reflector separation) than in (a) results in a large amplitude dip so that the echo pulses can be easily resolved, even with poor contrast resolution. (c) With overlap intermediate between (a) and (b), a moderate amplitude dip occurs. This may or may not be detected (depending on the contrast resolution [Section 4.4] of the instrument). Therefore, these echoes (and the reflectors from which they originated) may or may not be resolved on the display.

3.5.7 Doubling the frequency causes axial resolution to be _____.

3.5.8 Doubling the number of cycles per pulse causes axial resolution to be _____.

3.5.9 When studying an obese subject, a higher frequency will likely be required. True or false?

3.5.10 If better resolution is desired, a lower frequency will help. True or false?

3.5.11 If frequencies less than ____ MHz are used, axial resolution is not sufficient.

3.5.12 If frequencies higher than ____ MHz are used, half-intensity depth is not sufficient.

3.5.13 Increasing the frequency improves resolution because _____ is reduced, thus reducing _____ _____.

3.5.14 Increasing the frequency decreases the half-intensity depth because _____ is increased.

3.5.15 Lateral resolution is the minimum _____ between two

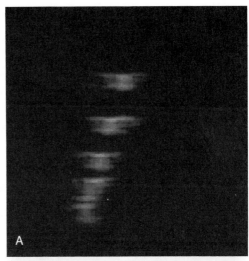

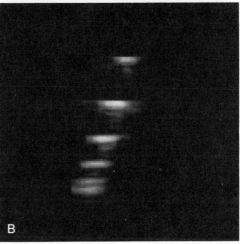

Figure 3.23. (a) An image of a set of six rods in the AIUM Test Object (Chapter 7). They are separated by 5, 4, 3, 2, and 1 mm from top to bottom. This scan was made using a transducer that produces ultrasound pulses at a frequency of 3.5 million cycles per second (i.e, a 3.5-MHz transducer). The first three rods have been separated, whereas the images of the last three rods have merged; therefore, the axial resolution is about 3 mm. This image also shows small reverberation echoes behind each image. These artifacts are discussed in Chapter 5. (b) The same rods imaged with a 5-MHz transducer. Higher frequency transducers produce shorter pulse lengths and therefore provide improved axial resolution.

reflectors such that when a beam is scanned across them, two separate _____ are produced.

3.5.16 Lateral resolution is equal to _____ _____.

3.5.17 Lateral resolution is also called (more than one correct answer)

    a. axial resolution

    b. longitudinal resolution

    c. angular resolution

    d. azimuthal resolution

    e. range resolution

    f. transverse resolution

    g. depth resolution

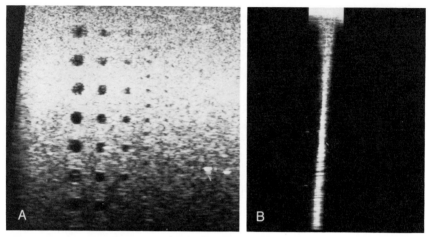

Figure 3.24. (a) An image of a resolution penetration phantom that contains circular anechoic regions ("cysts") in tissue-equivalent material (Chapter 7). From left to right, the "cysts" are 10, 8, 6, 4, 3, and 2 mm in diameter and occur every 1 to 2 cm in the depth of the field. Close examination shows that the 3-mm "cysts" are the smallest that can be resolved, and they are visible only in the range of 5 to 11 cm depth. This image was produced using a 3.5-MHz transducer. The beam profile of this transducer is shown in (b). From this image, the focus appears to be at about 8 cm depth.

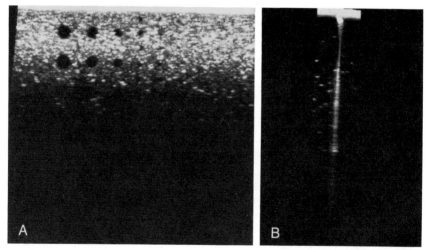

Figure 3.25. (a) The same phantom as in Figure 3.24(a) imaged with a 7.5-MHz transducer. In this instance, the 2-mm "cysts" can be seen in the first 4 cm of depth. This corresponds to the focal region of this transducer, as shown in its beam profile (b). Also note in (a) that the imaging depth is substantially reduced compared with Figure 3.24(a). This reduction in imaging depth is due to the fact that the tissue attenuation increases with increasing frequency (3 MHz to 7.5 MHz). Detail resolution can be improved by increasing the frequency of the ultrasound beam, but at the expense of decreasing the image depth.

3.5.18 For a transducer of given diameter, increasing the frequency improves lateral resolution. True or false?

3.5.19 Lateral resolution varies with distance from the transducer. True or false?

3.5.20 For a given frequency, a smaller transducer always gives improved lateral resolution. True or false?

3.5.21 Lateral resolution is determined by (more than one correct answer)
- a. damping
- b. frequency
- c. transducer diameter
- d. number of cycles in the pulse
- e. distance from transducer
- f. focusing

3.6
Review

Transducers convert energy from one form to another. Ultrasound transducers convert electric energy to ultrasound energy and vice versa. They operate on the piezoelectricity principle. Transducers may be operated in continuous mode or pulsed mode. Axial resolution is equal to one half the spatial pulse length. Pulsed transducers have damping material to shorten the spatial pulse length. Disc transducers produce sound in the form of beams with near and far zones. Lateral resolution is equal to beam diameter. Beam diameter may be reduced by focusing. Definitions of terms discussed in this chapter are listed below:

Annular array. Array made up of ring-shaped elements arranged concentrically.

Array. Transducer array.

Axial. In the direction of the transducer axis (sound-travel direction).

Axial resolution. Minimum reflector separation along the sound path required for separate reflections to be produced.

Bandwidth. Range of frequencies contained in an ultrasound pulse.

Continuous mode. Continuous-wave mode.

Damping. Material placed behind the rear face of a transducer element to reduce pulse duration; also, the process of pulse duration reduction.

Disc. Thin flat circular object.

Electric voltage. Electric potential or potential difference expressed in volts.

Far zone. The region of a sound beam in which the beam diameter increases as the distance from the transducer increases.

Focal length. Distance from focused transducer to center of focal region or to the location of the spatial peak intensity.

Focal region. Region of minimum beam diameter and area.

Focus. To concentrate the sound beam into a smaller beam area than would exist otherwise.

Fractional bandwidth. Bandwidth divided by operating frequency.

Grating lobes. Additional minor beams of sound traveling out in directions different from the primary beam. These result from the multielement structure of transducer arrays.

Internal focus. A focus produced by a curved transducer element.

Lateral. Perpendicular to the direction of sound travel.

Lateral resolution. Minimum reflector separation perpendicular to the sound path required for separate reflections to be produced.

Linear array. Array made up of rectangular elements in a line.

Linear phased array. Linear array operated by applying voltage pulses to all elements, but with small time differences.

Linear switched array. Linear array operated by applying voltage pulses to groups of elements sequentially.

Matching layer. Material placed in front of the front face of a transducer element to reduce the reflection at the transducer surface.

Near zone. The region of a sound beam in which the beam diameter decreases as the distance from the transducer increases.

Operating frequency. Preferred frequency of operation of a transducer.

Piezoelectricity. Conversion of pressure to electric voltage.

Probe. Transducer assembly.

Pulsed mode. Mode of operation in which pulsed ultrasound is used.

Quality factor. Operating frequency divided by bandwidth.

Resonance frequency. Operating frequency.

Sensitivity. Ability of an imaging system to detect weak reflections.

Side lobes. Minor beams of sound traveling out in directions different from the primary beam.

Sound beam. The region of a medium that contains virtually all the sound produced by a transducer.

Transducer. Device that converts energy from one form to another.

Transducer array. Transducer assembly containing more than one transducer element.

Transducer assembly. Transducer element and damping and matching materials assembled in a case.

Transducer element. Piece of piezoelectric material in a transducer assembly.

Ultrasound transducer. Device that converts electric energy to ultrasound energy and vice versa.

Voltage pulse. Brief excursion of voltage from its normal value.

Exercises

3.6.1 Match the following transducer assembly parts with their functions:
   a. cable: _____   1. reduces reflection at
   b. damping material: _____   transducer surface
   c. piezoelectric element: _____   2. converts voltage pulses
   d. matching layer: _____   to sound pulses
                                         3. reduces pulse duration
                                         4. conducts voltage pulses

3.6.2 Which of the following improve sound transmission from the transducer element into the tissue? (More than one correct answer.)
   a. matching layer
   b. doppler effect
   c. damping material
   d. coupling medium
   e. refraction

3.6.3 A transducer has a thickness of 0.4 mm, a diameter of 13 mm, and an element material propagation speed of 4 mm/μs. Calculate the following:
   a. operating frequency: _____ MHz
   b. wavelength in soft tissue: _____ mm
   c. near-zone length in soft tissue: _____ mm
   d. lateral resolution at 14 cm: _____ mm
   e. lateral resolution at 28 cm: _____ mm

3.6.4 Lateral resolution is improved by
   a. damping
   b. pulsing
   c. focusing
   d. reflecting
   e. absorbing

3.6.5 For an unfocused transducer, the best lateral resolution (minimum beam diameter) is _____ times the transducer diameter. This value of lateral resolution is found at a distance from the transducer face equal to the _____ length.

3.6.6 For a focused transducer, the best lateral resolution (minimum beam diameter) is found in the _____ region.

3.6.7 An unfocused 3.5-MHz 13-mm in diameter transducer will give a minimum beam diameter (best lateral resolution) of _____ mm.

3.6.8 An unfocused 3.5-MHz 13-mm in diameter transducer produces pulses of 3 cycles. The axial resolution in soft tissue is _____ mm.

3.6.9 In Exercises 3.6.7 and 3.6.8, axial resolution is better than lateral resolution. True or false?

3.6.10 Axial resolution is often not as good as lateral resolution in diagnostic ultrasound. True or false?

3.6.11 The two resolutions may be comparable in the _____ region of a highly focused beam.

3.6.12 Beam diameter may be reduced in the near zone by focusing. True or false?

3.6.13 Beam diameter may be reduced in the far zone by focusing. True or false?

3.6.14 Match each transducer characteristic with the sound beam characteristic it determines (answers may be used more than once):
    a. element thickness: ____, ____, and ____. 1. axial resolution
    b. element diameter: ____   2. lateral
    c. element shape (flat or curved): ____   resolution
    d. damping: ____   3. operating
                                    frequency

3.6.15 The axial resolution of a transducer can be improved most by
    a. increasing the damping
    b. increasing the diameter
    c. decreasing the damping
    d. decreasing the frequency
    e. decreasing the diameter
    f. attaching a doppler

3.6.16 The principle on which ultrasound transducers operate is the
    a. doppler effect
    b. acousto-optic effect
    c. acoustoelectric effect
    d. cause and effect
    e. piezoelectric effect

3.6.17 Which of the following is *not* decreased by damping?
    a. refraction
    b. pulse duration
    c. spatial pulse length
    d. efficiency
    e. sensitivity

3.6.18 Which three things determine beam diameter for a disc transducer?
    a. pulse duration
    b. frequency
    c. disc diameter
    d. distance from disc face
    e. efficiency

3.6.19 A two-cycle pulse of 5-MHz ultrasound produces separate reflections from reflectors in soft tissue separated by 1 mm. True or false?

3.6.20 The lower and upper limits of the frequency range useful in diagnostic ultrasound are determined by _____ and _____ _____ requirements, respectively.

3.6.21 The range of frequencies useful for diagnostic ultrasound is ____ to ____ MHz.

3.6.22 Because diagnostic ultrasound pulses are usually two or three cycles long, axial resolution is usually equal to _____ or _____ wavelengths.

3.6.23 What is the axial resolution in Figure 3.23(b)?

3.6.24 The best lateral resolution in Figure 3.13(c) is at what depth?

3.6.25 At the bottom of Figure 3.13(c) (15 cm depth) the pulse width is about 1 cm. What is the pulse width at the focus?

Chapter 4

Imaging Instruments

4.1
Introduction

In the preceding chapters the process by which ultrasound is generated and how it interacts with tissues were described. The instruments that detect and present the information resulting from this interaction will now be considered. The pulse-echo method (Figs. 1.1, 1.2, and 4.1) uses received echoes. This method consists of ultrasound generation, propagation, and reflection in tissues and reception of returning reflections. Most diagnostic ultrasound systems in use today are the reflection (pulse-echo) type. These instruments detect three things: the strength, direction, and arrival time of reflections that occur in the tissues. This chapter describes what the instruments do with these quantities.

Imaging systems produce visual displays from the electric voltages received from the transducer. A diagram of the components of a pulse-echo imaging system is given in Figure 4.2. Several parameters that describe ultrasound were given in Chapters 2 and 3. They are determined in this system as shown in Table 4.1.

In this chapter we consider the following questions: How do ultrasound imaging instruments work? What are the primary components in an instrument? What is the purpose of time gain compensation (TGC)? How are images stored electronically? What is contrast resolution and on what does it depend? How do displays work? What are the common display modes in imaging? The following terms are discussed in this chapter:

A mode   amplifier
amplification   analog

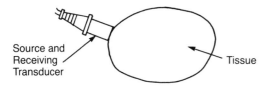

Source and
Receiving
Transducer

Tissue

Figure 4.1. Diagnostic ultrasound pulse-echo information collection method. This method responds to reflection, attenuation, and propagation speed encountered in the tissue.

B mode
B scan
bistable
bistable display
bit
cathode ray tube
compensation
compression
demodulation
digital
dynamic focusing
dynamic imaging
dynamic range
frame
frame rate

gain
gray scale
gray-scale display
gray-scale resolution
M mode
pixel
real-time
real-time display
rejection
scan converters
scan line
scanning
TGC
variable focusing

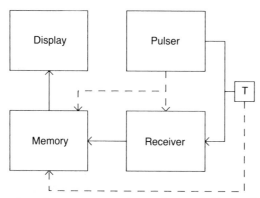

Display

Pulser

T

Memory

Receiver

Figure 4.2. The components of a pulse-echo imaging system. The pulser produces electric pulses (Figure 4.3) that drive the transducer (T). It also produces pulses that tell the receiver and memory when the transducer has been driven. The transducer (acting as a source) produces an ultrasound pulse (Figure 4.3) for each electric pulse applied. For each reflection received from the tissues, an electric voltage is produced by the transducer (acting as a receiving transducer). These voltages go to the receiver, where they are processed to a form suitable for driving the memory. Information on transducer orientation (which way it is pointing) is delivered (dashed lines) by electric voltages to the memory. Electric information from memory drives the display, which produces a visual image of the cross-sectional anatomy interrogated by the system. Some authors consider a clock or timing circuit separately in a diagram such as this. The clock determines the pulse repetition frequency and causes the various components of the instrument to work together. In this figure and in Sections 4.1 and 4.2, the clock is considered to be part of the pulser.

Table 4.1
Determination of Ultrasound Parameters*

Ultrasound Parameter	Determined by
Frequency	transducer
Period	transducer
Wavelength	transducer, tissue
Propagation speed	tissue
Pulse repetition frequency	pulser
Pulse repetition period	pulser
Pulse duration	transducer
Duty factor	pulser, transducer
Spatial pulse length	transducer, tissue
Axial resolution	transducer, tissue
Amplitude	pulser, transducer
Intensity	pulser, transducer
Attenuation	transducer, tissue
Half-intensity depth	transducer, tissue
Beam diameter	transducer, tissue
Lateral resolution	transducer, tissue

*The ultrasound parameters described in Chapters 2 and 3 are determined by imaging system components described in Chapters 3 and 4 (Fig. 4.2). Overall imaging system axial and lateral resolutions are also determined by the receiver, memory, and display.

Exercises

4.1.1 The five primary components of a diagnostic ultrasound imaging system are the _____, _____, _____, _____, and _____.

4.1.2 Match each component with its function:

a. pulser: _____ 1. produces ultrasound pulses
b. transducer: _____ 2. processes voltages received from the transducer
c. receiver: _____
d. memory: _____ 3. receives electrical information from the memory
e. display: _____
4. produces electrical pulses that drive the transducer
5. provides electrical information to the display

4.1.3 Match these ultrasound parameters produced by an instrument with the components that determine them (answers may be used more than once):

a. frequency: _____   1. pulser
b. period: _____   2. transducer
c. wavelength: _____, _____   3. tissue
d. propagation speed: _____
e. pulse repetition frequency: _____
f. pulse repetition period: _____
g. pulse duration: _____
h. duty factor: _____
i. spatial pulse length: _____, _____
j. axial resolution: _____, _____
k. amplitude: _____, _____
l. intensity: _____, _____
m. attenuation: _____, _____
n. half-intensity depth: _____, _____
o. beam diameter: _____, _____
p. lateral resolution: _____, _____

4.2
Pulser

The pulser is where the action originates. It produces electric voltage pulses (Fig. 4.3) that (1) drive the transducer, which produces ultrasound pulses, and (2) tell the receiver and memory when the ultrasound pulses are produced. The pulse repetition frequency of the pulse is the number of electric pulses produced per second. It is typically 1000 Hz or 1 kHz. The ultrasound pulse repetition frequency is equal to the voltage pulse repetition frequency, since one ultrasound pulse is produced for each voltage pulse (Fig. 4.3). Similarly, the ultrasound pulse repetition period is equal to the voltage pulse repetition period. The voltage pulse duration is much less than the period of the cycles in the ultrasound pulses. To receive information for display at a rapid rate, it is necessary to use a high repetition frequency. Repetition frequency, however, must be limited in order to provide an unambiguous display of returning reflections. This is described in Chapter 5. The timing sequence that is initiated by the pulse is shown in Figure 4.4.

Included in the functions of the pulser, in which array transducers are used, is the production of delays and variations in pulse amplitudes

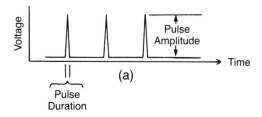

(a)

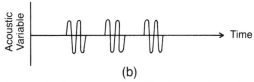

(b)

Figure 4.3. An ultrasound pulse (b) is produced by the transducer for every voltage pulse (a) applied.

necessary for the electronic control of beam scanning, steering, and shaping described in Section 3.4. Suppression of grating lobes is accomplished, as well, by a process called dynamic apodization. In this, electric pulse amplitudes are adjusted for the various array elements in order to suppress grating lobes and improve the dynamic range (discussed in Section 4.3) of the system. All of this is accomplished by what is sometimes called a digital beam former. It is considered here to be part of the pulser. It is called digital because it performs these functions under computer control.

The greater the pulse amplitude produced by the pulser, the greater

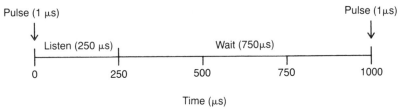

Time (μs)

Figure 4.4. Timing sequence for pulse echo ultrasound imaging. The sequence is initiated by the production of a 1-μs pulse of ultrasound when the pulser sends a voltage pulse to the transducer. This is followed by a period of up to 250 μs during which echoes are received from the tissue by the transducer. The length of this time is determined by the maximum depth from which the echoes return. For example, for 2 MHz, echoes can return from as deep as 20 cm. The round-trip travel time to this depth is 260 ms. This listening period is followed by a waiting period until the next pulse is produced. In this illustration, the waiting period is 750 μs. Here, the pulse repetition period is 1000 μs (pulse repetition frequency, 1 kHz). If the pulse repetition frequency were greater, the pulse repetition period would be less, resulting in a shorter waiting period.

Table 4.2
Ranges for Acoustic Output Parameters of
Diagnostic Ultrasound Imaging Instruments[13-16]

Parameter	Range
SATA intensity	0.06–60 mW/cm^2
SPTA intensity	0.01–200 mW/cm^2
SPPA intensity	0.5–280 W/cm^2
Beam uniformity ratio	
Unfocused	2–3
Focused	5–200
Duty factor	0.001–0.003
Cycles per pulse	2–6
Pulse repetition frequency	0.5–3 kHz

will be the amplitude and intensity of the ultrasound pulses produced by the transducer. Ultrasound pulse amplitude and intensity depend also on the transducer efficiency. Electric pulse amplitudes are generally a few tens or hundreds of volts. Table 4.2 gives typical ranges for acoustic outputs of diagnostic instruments.

Exercises

4.2.1 The ultrasound pulse repetition frequency is equal to the voltage _____ repetition frequency of the pulser.

4.2.2 Increased pulse amplitude produced by the pulser increases the _____ and _____ of ultrasound pulses produced by the transducer.

4.2.3 Match these acoustic parameters produced by diagnostic instruments with their typical values:

a. SATA intensity: _____   1. 50

b. SPPA intensity: _____   2. 0.001

c. beam uniformity ratio: _____   3. 1 mW/cm^2

d. duty factor: _____   4. 3

e. cycles per pulse: _____   5. 1 W/cm^2

4.3
Receiver

Voltages produced in the transducer by returning reflections are sent to the receiver for processing. The receiver performs the following functions:

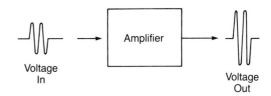

Figure 4.5. Amplification increases voltage amplitude and electric power.

1. amplification
2. compensation
3. compression
4. demodulation
5. rejection

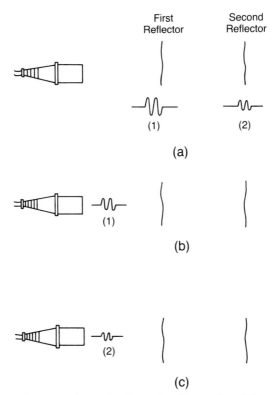

Figure 4.6. Two reflectors with equal reflection coefficients but different distances from the transducer. (a) The reflected pulse at the second reflector is weaker because the incident pulse has to travel farther to get to the second reflector, thus experiencing more attenuation. (b) The reflection from the first reflector arrives at the transducer. It is weaker than it was in (a) because of attenuation on the return trip. (c) The reflection from the second reflector arrives at the transducer later and weaker than the first one did. This is because of the longer path to the second reflector.

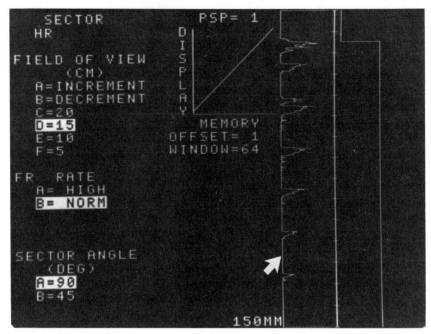

Figure 4.7. This display shows an amplitude-mode (Section 4.5) presentation of the metal-rod echoes in Figure 1.3. The vertical line (arrow) represents depth from top to bottom. The deflections to the right indicate the amplitudes of the echoes from the rods. It is seen that echo amplitude decreases with depth even though reflection coefficients for all the rods are the same. The decreasing amplitude is a result of increasing attenuation for the longer paths to the deeper rods.

Amplification is increasing the small voltages received from the transducer to larger ones suitable for processing and storage (Fig. 4.5). Gain is the ratio of output to input electric power. The power ratio is equal to the square of the voltage ratio (across the same resistance); power ratio may be expressed in decibels (Appendix C). For example, if the input voltage amplitude to an amplifier is 2 mV and the output voltage amplitude is 200 mV, the voltage ratio is 200/2 or 100. The power ratio is $(100)^2$ or 10,000. From Table C.2 (Appendix C) the power ratio of gain is found to be 40 dB. Receiver amplifiers usually have 60 to 100 dB of gain. Voltages applied to these amplifiers range from tens of microvolts to tens of millivolts.

Compensation (also called gain compensation, swept gain, time gain compensation [TGC], or depth gain compensation) equalizes differences in received reflection amplitudes because of reflector depth. Reflectors with equal reflection coefficients (Section 2.5) will not result in equal amplitude reflections arriving at the transducer (Figs. 4.6 and 4.7) if their travel distances are different (distances from the transducer to the

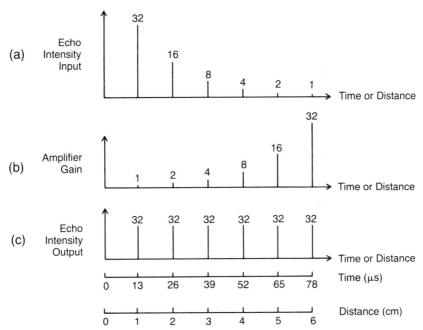

Figure 4.8. Compensation of attenuation by varying amplification. The time scale represents the arrival time of reflections. The distance scale represents the distance from the transducer to the reflectors. (a) Arriving reflections produce different echo intensities because of attenuation. All reflections are assumed here to have come from reflectors with equal reflection coefficients. Each reflection arrives 13 μs after the previous one, and thus for soft tissue each reflector is 1 cm farther from the transducer (Exercise 2.5.47). Each reflection produces an echo intensity one half that of the previous one in this example. (b) Amplification must compensate for this by doubling as each 13 μs of time passes during the arrival of the reflections. Each arriving echo intensity (a) times the gain or amplification (b) existing at the time the voltage arrives at the amplifier equals the echo intensity out of the amplifier (c). Following this process, all the intensities are equalized. This is the case where all reflections result from equal reflection coefficients. If reflection coefficients of the various reflectors are different, the resulting echo intensities, even after compensation, will be different. These differences should not be normalized or information would be lost.

reflectors are different). This is because attenuation depends on path length (Section 2.4). It is desirable to display reflections from reflectors of equal reflection coefficients, sizes, and shapes in a similar way. As these reflections may not arrive with the same amplitude, because of different path lengths, their amplitudes must be adjusted to compensate for path length differences. Larger path lengths result in later arrival times. Therefore, if voltages from reflections arriving later are amplified more than earlier ones, attenuation compensation is accomplished. This is what compensation does (Figs. 4.8 and 4.9).

The rate of increase of gain with depth is commonly called the TGC slope because it is often displayed graphically as a line with increasing

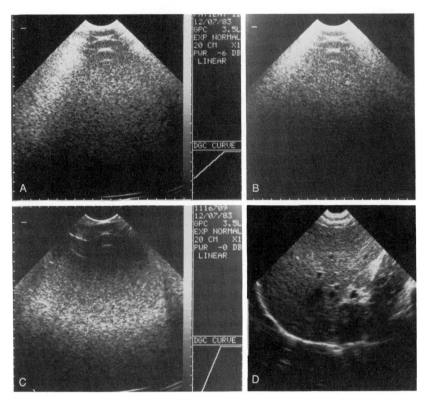

Figure 4.9. Three scans of a tissue-equivalent phantom imaged at 3.5 MHz with different settings of the time gain compensation (TGC). These scans show (a) correct compensation, (b) undercompensation, and (c) overcompensation. (d) shows a liver scan with proper TGC. Without TGC, the echo brightness (amplitude, intensity, strength) would fall off with depth (top to bottom).

height (lower right-hand corners of Fig. 4.9a, b, and c). This slope is expressed in decibels (gain) per centimeter depth. When properly adjusted, the slope should correspond to the attenuation in the tissue in decibels per centimeter depth. Remember that each centimeter of depth corresponds to 2 cm of sound travel (Section 2.5), so that the resulting slope should be about 1 dB/cm-MHz. The slope in Figure 4.8 is 3 dB (doubling) per centimeter—i.e., the attenuation coefficient is 1.5 dB/cm (thus, the frequency is approximately 3 MHz). Because the attenuation depends upon the frequency of the ultrasound beam, the TGC is simultaneously adjusted by the operator to match the frequency as well as the tissues being imaged.

Compression is the process of decreasing the differences between the smallest and largest amplitudes (Fig. 4.10). This is accomplished by

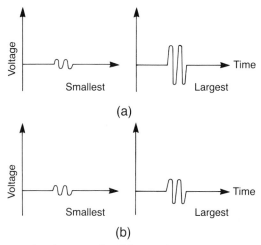

Figure 4.10. Compression decreases the difference between the smallest and largest voltage amplitudes passing through the system. (a) Before compression, the ratio of largest to smallest amplitudes is five. (b) After compression, the ratio is three.

logarithmic amplifiers that amplify weak inputs more than strong ones. The ratio of the largest power to the smallest power that the system can handle is called the dynamic range. It is expressed in decibels. For example, if an amplifier is insensitive to voltage amplitudes less than 0.01 mV and cannot properly handle voltage amplitudes greater than 1000 mV, the ratio of voltages is 1000/0.01 or 100,000. The power ratio is equal to the square of the voltage ratio: $(100,000)^2$ or 10,000,000,000. According to Table C.2 (Appendix C), the dynamic range of the amplifier is 100 dB. Although amplifiers have such a dynamic range (typically 100 to 120 dB), demodulators and displays do not. Their dynamic ranges are

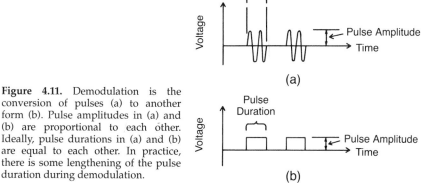

Figure 4.11. Demodulation is the conversion of pulses (a) to another form (b). Pulse amplitudes in (a) and (b) are proportional to each other. Ideally, pulse durations in (a) and (b) are equal to each other. In practice, there is some lengthening of the pulse duration during demodulation.

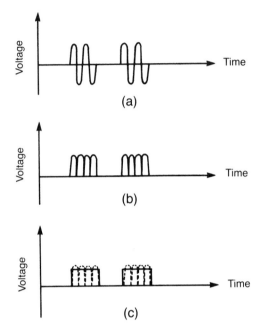

Figure 4.12. Rectification (b) and smoothing (filtering) (c) of pulses (a) results in demodulation (see Figure 4.11).

approximately 50 and 20 dB, respectively. The largest power can be only 100 times the smallest for the display. Thus, the largest voltage amplitude can only be 10 times the smallest. The dynamic range remaining after compensation is typically 40 to 50 dB. A compressor would have to compress the intensity ratio (100,000) corresponding to 50 dB to an intensity ratio of 100 (acceptable for the display).

Demodulation (sometimes called detection or envelope detection) is the process of converting the voltages delivered to the receiver from one form to another (Fig. 4.11). This is done by rectification and smoothing (filtering) (Fig. 4.12). Because diagnostic ultrasound pulses do not have constant amplitude (Fig. 2.15), when demodulated they do not have the blocked appearance shown in Figures 4.11 to 4.14 but rather appear as in Figure 3.22.

Rejection (sometimes called suppression or threshold) eliminates the smaller amplitude voltage pulses produced by weaker reflections or electronic noise (Fig. 4.13). The weaker reflections often come from side lobes or multiple scattering from within the tissue, thus constituting "acoustic noise." It is desirable to eliminate noise, electronic or acoustic, from the image, because it contributes no useful information and interferes with the observation of the useful information that *is* presented.

Figure 4.14 summarizes the five receiver functions discussed. The

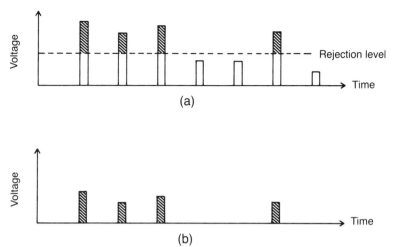

Figure 4.13. Rejection eliminates voltage pulses with amplitudes below the rejection level. (a) Before rejection. (b) After rejection.

amplification (gain), compensation, and rejection functions are normally operator-adjustable; demodulation and compression are not. Included in the functions of the receiver, in which phased-array transducers are used, is the insertion of appropriate delays in the voltages returning from the array and representing arriving echoes. This is done in order to accomplish the dynamic focusing discussed in Section 3.4.

Exercises

4.3.1 Five functions performed by the receiver are _____, _____, _____, _____, and _____.

4.3.2 Match the following functions with what they accomplish:
   a. amplification: _____   1. converts pulses from one form to
   b. compensation: _____   another
   c. compression: _____   2. increases all amplitudes
   d. demodulation: _____   3. decreases dynamic range
   e. rejection: _____   4. eliminates some pulses
                                 5. corrects for tissue attenuation

4.3.3 Input voltage to an amplifier is 1 mV and output voltage is 10 mV. The voltage amplification ratio is _____. The power ratio is _____. The gain is _____ dB.

4.3.4 A receiver with a gain of 60 dB has 1 μW of power applied to the input. The output power is _____ W.

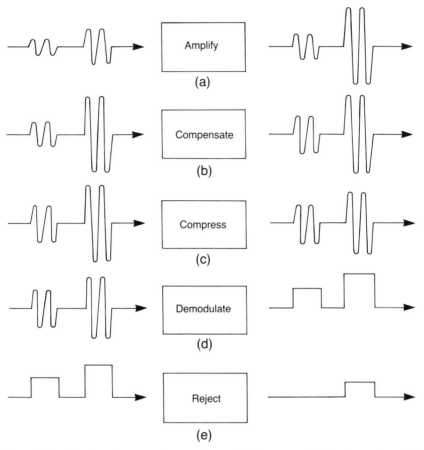

Figure 4.14. Five functions a receiver performs. The larger-amplitude pulse arrives first. (a) Both pulses are amplified, doubling their amplitudes in this example. (b) The latter (weaker) pulse is amplified more. (c) The difference between the pulse amplitudes is reduced. (d) The pulses are converted to another form. (e) The weaker pulse is rejected because it is not above the rejection level.

4.3.5 A receiver with a gain of 60 dB has 10 μV of voltage applied to the input. The output voltage is _____ mV.

4.3.6 Compensation is also called (more than one correct answer):
 a. swept beam
 b. swept gain
 c. refraction
 d. diffraction
 e. time gain compensation

4.3.7 Compensation takes into account reflector _____ or
_____.

4.3.8 Compensation amplifies pulses differently, according to their arrival _____.

4.3.9 Compression decreases the _____ range to a range that the _____ can handle.

4.3.10 If a display has a dynamic range of 20 dB and the smallest voltage it can handle is 200 mV, the largest voltage it can handle is _____ V.

4.3.11 Demodulation converts voltage _____ from one form to another.

4.3.12 Rejection eliminates higher-amplitude pulses. True or false?

4.3.13 Another name for rejection is
a. threshold
b. depth gain compensation
c. swept gain
d. compression
e. demodulation

4.4
Memory

Storing each cross-sectional image in memory as the sound beam is scanned through the tissue permits display of a single image (scan) out of the rapid sequence of several images (frames) normally acquired each second in dynamic (real-time) ultrasound instruments. Displaying one scan out of the sequence is called freeze-frame. Some instruments have enough memory to store the last several frames acquired. This is sometimes called "cine-loop."

Two types of image memories are used in diagnostic ultrasound instruments—analog and digital. These memories are commonly called scan converters because they provide a means for displaying, using a television scan format (Section 4.5), information acquired by a linear, sector, or other scanning technique (Section 4.5). The image plane is divided into squares called pixels (picture elements), commonly 1000 x 1000 or 2000 x 2000 (analog), 512 x 512 (square format digital), or 512 x 640 (rectangular format digital) squares on a side. In each of these spaces an electric charge (analog) or a number (digital) is stored that corresponds to the echo intensity received from the point within the body corresponding to that storage position.

The analog scan converter consists of a square matrix of electrical insulators, 1000 or 2000 on each side (1,000,000 or 4,000,000 total). An

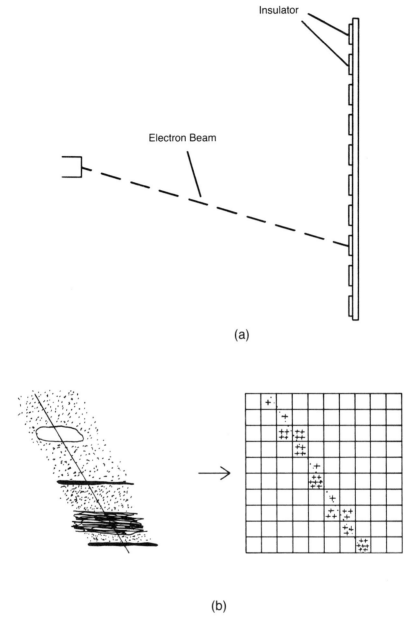

(a)

(b)

Figure 4.15. Analog scan converter. (a) Side view. A square matrix of insulators is scanned by an electron beam as the patient is scanned by the ultrasound beam. (b) Anatomic cross-section scanned and front view of scan converter. Electric charge is stored on the insulators in proportion to the intensity of the echoes received from corresponding anatomic locations.

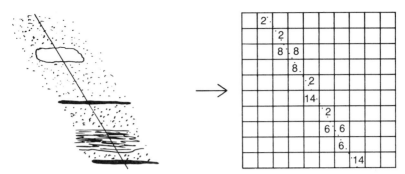

Figure 4.16. Anatomic cross-section scanned and front view of digital scan converter. Numbers are stored in the memory elements according to the intensity of the echoes received from corresponding anatomic locations.

electron beam is directed toward this matrix (Fig. 4.15a) and is swept across it in a direction corresponding to the direction in which the ultrasound passes through the body part (Fig. 4.15b). The current in the electron beam is increased and decreased, corresponding to the increasing and decreasing intensity of the series of echoes that comes back to the transducer as the transmitted ultrasound pulse travels through the tissue. This results in various electric charge strengths being stored in the individual storage elements of the analog scan converter. After a single ultrasound pulse has traveled through the tissue in a given path, the information corresponding to the returned echoes is stored along a corresponding path in the scan converter in the form of various electric charge values in the insulator elements along that path (Fig. 4.15b).

A digital scan converter is a computer memory that stores numbers. As in the analog scan converter, a matrix of digital memory elements is used to store echo information. Either a square matrix, 512 on a side (262,144 total), or a rectangular matrix, 512 x 640 (327,680 total), is used. In each of these elements a number is stored corresponding to the echo intensity received from the point within the body corresponding to that storage position (Fig. 4.16). If the digital memory were made up of a single matrix checkerboard, each pixel could only store one of two numbers, a zero or a one. This is because such memories are binary in nature and can only operate in two conditions, on or off, corresponding to one or zero. This would allow bistable or black and white imaging. In order to image gray scale (several shades of gray or brightness in addition to black and white), it is necessary to have more than one checkerboard. In a four-bit (binary digit) memory there are four checkerboards back to back so that each pixel has four bits associated with it. In the binary numbering system (Appendix C) this allows numbers from 0 to 15 (16-shade system) to be stored. Other examples are given in Table 4.3. A 10 x

Table 4.3
Characteristics of Digital Memories

Number of	Lowest Number Stored		Highest Number Stored		Number
Bits	DECIMAL	BINARY	DECIMAL	BINARY	of Shades
4	0	0000	15	1111	16
5	0	0000	31	11111	32
6	0	0000	63	111111	64
7	0	0000	127	1111111	128
8	0	0000	255	11111111	256

10, four-bit (per pixel) memory is shown in Figure 4.17. The total number of memory elements in various digital memories is given in Table 4.4.

The procedure for storing the information required for display of the two-dimensional cross-sectional image for either analog or digital scan converters is as follows: the beam is scanned through the patient in such a way that the ultrasound beam "cuts" through the tissue in cross section. Echoes received from all points on this cross section are converted to electric charges or numbers, which are stored at corresponding places in the analog or digital memory. All the information necessary for displaying this cross-sectional image is then stored in memory. The information can then be taken out of memory and applied to a two-dimensional display (cathode ray tube; Section 4.5) and displayed in such a way that the electric charge values or numbers coming out of memory are displayed with corresponding brightnesses on the face of the tube (Fig. 4.18). An example of such a display is shown in Figure 4.19.

Analog is derived from the Greek for "proportionate" and digital from Latin for "finger" or "toe." Analog scan converters are continuous in nature—that is, they can store any value of charge in each pixel from the minimum to the maximum capability of the device. Digital scan converters are discrete—that is, they can only store whole numbers in each

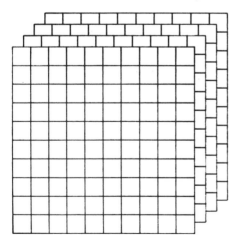

Figure 4.17. A 10 x 10 pixel, four-bit deep (4 bits per pixel) digital memory.

Table 4.4
Bits (Binary Digits or Memory Elements) in
Digital Memories

Dimensions	Pixels	Bits Deep	Total Bits
512 x 512	262,144	4	1,050,000
512 x 512	262,144	5	1,310,000
512 x 512	262,144	6	1,570,000
512 x 512	262,144	7	1,840,000
512 x 640	327,680	4	1,310,000
512 x 640	327,680	5	1,640,000
512 x 640	327,680	6	1,970,000
512 x 640	327,680	7	2,290,000

pixel location from zero to a maximum that is determined by the number of bits per pixel (Table 4.3).

For a 1000 x 1000 memory matrix in which the represented anatomic depth is 20 cm, each pixel represents anatomic dimensions of 0.2 mm. For a 512 x 512 matrix the result is 0.4 mm. This represents the spatial resolution of the memory matrix. If the maximum depth represented in memory is 10 cm, then the memory spatial resolutions are 0.1 and 0.2 mm, respectively. The 512 x 640 rectangular matrix is sometimes used because it is more representative of the oval shape of the normal abdomen cross section, in which the anterior-posterior dimension is about 80 per cent of the lateral dimension.

Preprocessing, in digital systems, is the assignment of specific numbers to echo intensities as they are stored in memory (Fig. 4.20). Postprocessing is the assignment of specific display brightnesses to numbers coming out of memory (Fig. 4.21). For most digital systems, the preprocessing scheme is a linear one (Fig. 4.20) and cannot be controlled by the operator. For a linear preprocessing assignment, the echo dynamic range is equally divided throughout the gray levels of the system. Table

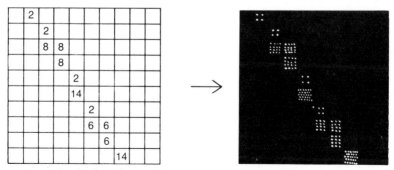

Figure 4.18. For display of scanned anatomic structures, numbers are read out of pixel locations in digital memory and applied to the display in such a way that brightness corresponds to stored number.

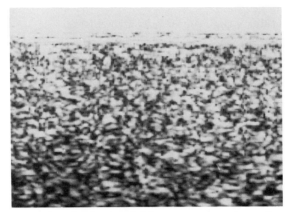

Figure 4.19. Display of pixels of various brightnesses representing various numbers in the corresponding memory locations. The display is magnified here to make the square pixels easily seen. Normally they are too small and numerous to be noticed individually.

4.5 gives, for four- to seven-bit systems, the number of decibels per shade (assuming a 40-dB echo dynamic range after attenuation compensation) and the average intensity difference between two echoes in order for them to be assigned to different shades (number in memory) in the system. This is known as contrast (gray-scale) resolution. For a four-bit sys-

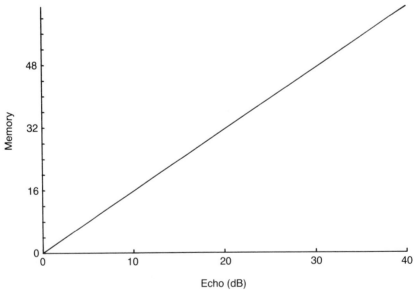

Figure 4.20. Digital preprocessing is the assignment of numbers (to be stored in memory) to echo intensities. Here echo intensity is expressed in decibels (relative to the weakest echo, which is represented as 0 dB; forty decibels is the strongest echo—10,000 times the intensity of the weakest).

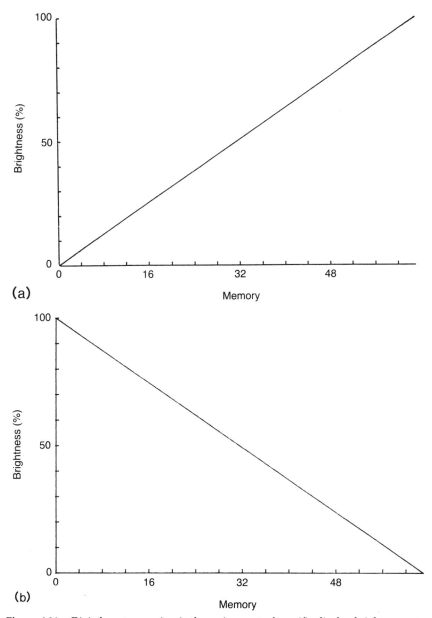

Figure 4.21. Digital postprocessing is the assignment of specific display brightnesses to numbers coming out of specific pixel locations in memory. (a) Increasing brightness with increasing echo intensity is seen. This is sometimes called a white-echo display. (b) Increasing brightness with decreasing echo intensity (black-echo display) is shown. Both forms of display were common in the early days of gray-scale imaging. The latter is now seldom used. Figure 4.7 (top center) shows such a postprocessing assignment on an instrument display.

Table 4.5
Contrast Resolution of Digital Memories*

Bits per Pixel	Decibels per Shade	Intensity Difference (%)[†]
4	2.5	78
5	1.2	32
6	0.6	15
7	0.3	7

*Assuming a 40-dB echo dynamic range.
†The average difference required between two echoes in order for them to be assigned to different shades.

tem, an echo must have nearly twice the intensity of another one for it to get assigned a different shade. For a seven-bit system, only a 7 per cent difference is required. On many instruments, one of several preprogrammed postprocessing schemes is selectable by the operator. On others, the postprocessing curve may be designed as desired by the operator using panel controls. A linear assignment (Fig. 4.21) equally divides the display brightness range among the stored gray levels of the system. Other schemes (Fig. 4.22) may be used that allow assignment of more of the brightness range to certain portions of the stored-number range capability of the system. Figure 4.22(a) represents one of the most useful schemes, which assigns more gray scale range to the weaker

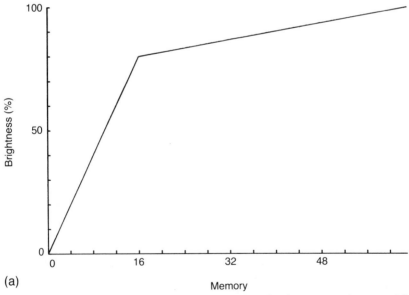

(a)

Figure 4.22. Postprocessing assignment schemes. A large brightness range is reserved for (a) weak, (b) strong, and (c) intermediate echoes.

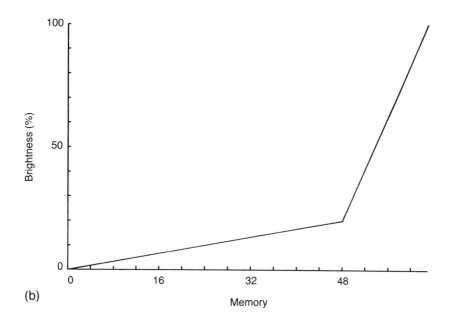

(b)

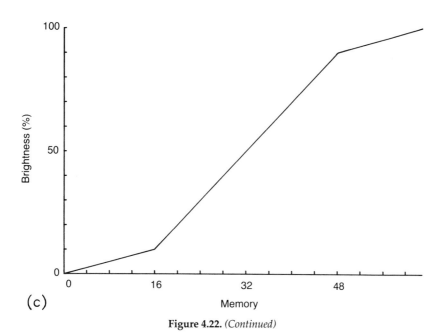

(c)

Figure 4.22. *(Continued)*

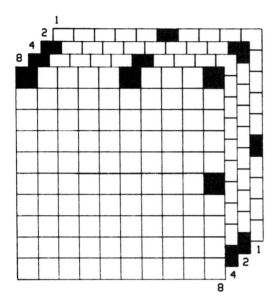

Figure 4.23. Digital memory description for Exercise 4.4.1. White indicates that the memory device is on.

echoes that result from scattering and are therefore angle-independent (Section 2.5).

Some digital instruments digitize the electric voltages coming out of the receiver. Some digitize earlier in the process, allowing some receiver functions to be carried out digitally, e.g., demodulation.

Exercises

4.4.1 For the digital memory shown in Figure 4.23, match pixel locations with numbers stored:
   a. lower right: _____   1. 13
   b. middle right: _____   2. 10
   c. upper right: _____   3. 9
   d. upper middle: _____   4. 14
   e. upper left: _____   5. 6

4.4.2 The contrast resolution for a digital instrument that has an echo dynamic range of 43 dB and 32 shades is _____ dB per shade.
   a. 1.3
   b. 3.2
   c. 4.3
   d. 32
   e. 43

4.4.3 The contrast resolution for a six-bit digital instrument that has an echo dynamic range of 45 dB is _____.

a. 0.3
b. 0.5
c. 0.7
d. 0.9
e. 6

4.4.4 Match the following:

a. analog: _____   1. picture element
b. digital: _____   2. assignment of stored numbers
c. preprocessing: _____   3. discrete
d. postprocessing: _____ 4. binary digit
e. pixel: _____   5. continuous
f. bit: _____   6. assignment of displayed
                             brightnesses

4.4.5 Typical digital pixel matrix dimensions are _____.

a. 640 x 128
b. 16 x 64
c. 100 x 100
d. 512 x 1540
e. 512 x 512

4.4.6 Match the number of shades with bits per pixel:

a. 16: _____   1. 1
b. 32: _____   2. 2
c. 64: _____   3. 3
d. 128: _____   4. 4
e. 256: _____   5. 5
                      6. 6
                      7. 7
                      8. 8
                      9. 9
                      10. 10

4.4.7 _____ total memory elements are required for a 100 x 100 pixel, five-bit digital memory.

4.4.8 Analog scan converters store information in terms of _____.

a. logarithms
b. electrical magnetism
c. electrical current
d. electrical charge
e. numbers

4.4.9 Digital scan converters store _____.

a. logarithms
b. electrical magnetism
c. electrical current
d. electrical charge
e. numbers

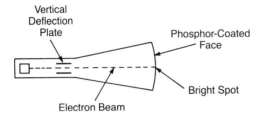

Figure 4.24 A cathode-ray tube (side view). The electron beam produces a bright spot where it strikes the phosphor-coated face of the tube. There is a set of horizontal deflection plates that is not shown.

4.4.10 _____ is commonly controllable by the operator.
  a. postprocessing
  b. contrast resolution
  c. bits per pixel
  d. digitalization
  e. all of the above

4.5
Display

There are several ways in which the information delivered to the display may be presented. Those in common use are:

1. A mode
2. B mode
3. M mode
4. B scan

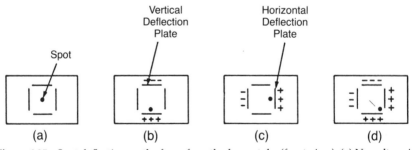

Figure 4.25 Spot deflection on the face of a cathode-ray tube (front view). (a) No voltage is applied to deflection plates; the spot is centered. (b) Voltage is applied to vertical deflection plates; the spot is deflected down. Increasing the voltage increases the deflection. If applied voltage were reversed, the spot would be deflected up. (c) Voltage is applied to horizontal deflection plates; the spot is deflected to the right. (d) Voltage is applied to both sets of plates; the spot is deflected down and to the right.

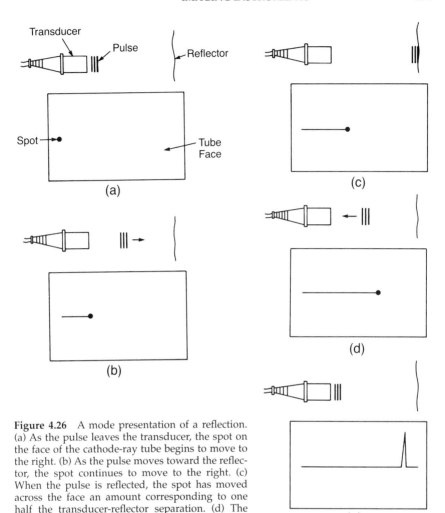

Figure 4.26 A mode presentation of a reflection. (a) As the pulse leaves the transducer, the spot on the face of the cathode-ray tube begins to move to the right. (b) As the pulse moves toward the reflector, the spot continues to move to the right. (c) When the pulse is reflected, the spot has moved across the face an amount corresponding to one half the transducer-reflector separation. (d) The spot continues to move to the right as the reflection moves toward the transducer. (e) When the reflection arrives at the transducer, an electric pulse is delivered to the receiver, which delivers an electric pulse to the display. This is applied to vertical deflection plates, causing the spot to deflect up at horizontal position corresponding to the transducer-reflector separation. This process is repeated each time a pulse is delivered from the pulser to the transducer. A system with no memory is assumed in this description. Memory is not necessary in A mode presentations.

The display device used in each case is a cathode ray tube. This tube generates a sharply focused beam of electrons that produces a bright spot on the phosphor-coated front face (screen) of the tube (Fig. 4.24). This spot can be moved across or up and down the face by applying voltages to deflection plates (Fig. 4.25) or electric currents to magnetic deflection coils. If the voltage or current is properly varied, the spot can be made to move across the face at constant speed. At the completion of this motion (i.e., when a scan line is completed), the spot can be made to jump rapidly back to the starting point.

Amplitude mode (A mode) operation causes a vertical deflection of the spot each time a pulse is delivered from the receiver (i.e., each time a reflection is received by the transducer). The horizontal position of the vertical deflection (Fig. 4.26) is determined by pulse travel time (and thus by reflector distance). The vertical deflection amplitude is determined by the received reflection amplitude and by the amplification, compensation, compression, and rejection of the receiver. The A mode is commonly used in setting up M mode presentations.

Brightness mode (B mode) operation causes a brightening of the spot rather than a deflection each time a reflection is received (Fig. 4.27). Back-and-forth motion of the reflector is seen as back-and-forth motion of the vertical deflection in the A mode or the bright spot in the B mode.

Motion mode (M mode) operation is B mode operation in which the motion of the spots is recorded by a recording medium (strip chart recorder) that moves across the face of the display. This results in a recording of the reflector motion (Fig. 4.27). The M mode is commonly used in heart studies.

B scan (B mode scan) operation causes a brightening of the spot, as in the B and M modes. However, the scan lines are not horizontal, as they are in the B and M modes. The starting point and direction of motion across the face are determined in the B mode by the starting point and direction of the beam. An image (B scan) of the object scanned may be built up on the face of the tube as the beam is moved through the tissue cross section (Figs. 1.4 to 1.7). Some means of storing echo information during this scanning must be provided. This was discussed in the previous section. The B scan is an image that is a cross section of the object through the scanning plane, as if the sound beam were cutting a section through the tissue. Figure 4.9 (d) is an example.

The A mode and M mode presentations discussed previously are one-dimensional and real-time in nature. It was shown, however, that producing the two-dimensional images of the B scan required scanning the beam. With a manual static scanning process, it is not possible to produce images rapidly enough to produce a display that continuously images moving structures (real-time display).

Figure 4.27. Three presentations of a reflection. Reflection 1 is produced at a stationary reflector. Reflection 2 is produced at a deeper reflector that is moving back and forth. (a) Vertical deflection 2 in the A mode moves left and right as the reflector moves close to and farther from the transducer. (b) The bright spot 2 in the B mode moves left and right as the reflector moves closer to and farther from the transducer. (c) As the process is repeated and a recording medium is moved across the face of the display, the motion of reflector 2 is traced out in the M mode.

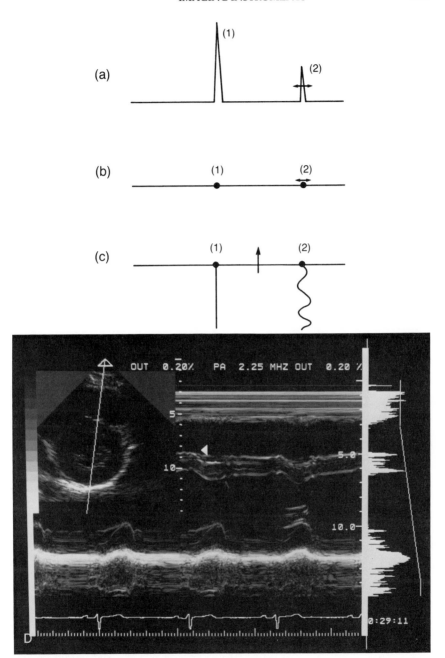

Figure 4.27. *(Continued)* (d) Clinical example of A and M modes with two-dimensional image superimposed at upper left; A mode is at right; M mode is at bottom and at upper center. The white line in the two-dimensional image indicates the scan line from which A and M mode presentations are derived. Short axis view of the cardiac left ventricle. (Courtesy of Advanced Technology Laboratories.)

Real-time or dynamic imaging instruments must produce several cross-sectional images per second. This requires the use of mechanical or array real-time transducers. Ten to 60 images are displayed per second (frame rate), yielding what appears to be a continuously changing image. Dynamic imaging instruments may or may not have a memory. Because the images are produced rapidly in sequence, memory is not required, as it is in the case of the manual scan, which takes a second or two to produce and then is observed for several seconds. If a real-time instrument has static-image (freeze-frame) capability, it must have a memory. Dynamic imaging provides rapid and convenient acquisition of the desired image (the display changes continuously as the beam is scanned through the tissues) and two-dimensional imaging of the motion of moving structures (the display continuously changes as the structures move).

Each complete scan of the sound beam produces an image on the display that is called a frame. Each frame is made of scan lines (one for each time the transducer is pulsed). The pulse repetition frequency needed is determined by the required lines per frame and the frame rate:

pulse repetition frequency (Hz) = lines per frame x frame rate

PRF = LPF x FR

lines per frame   ↑   pulse repetition frequency   ↑

frame rate   ↑   pulse repetition frequency   ↑

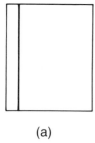

(a)

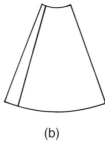

(b)

Figure 4.28 Rectangular (a) and sector (b) display formats for dynamic-imaging instruments. Linear switched or sequenced arrays produce a rectangular scan format (a) whereas mechanical real-time and phased array transducers produce a sector scan format (b). (From Kremkau, F.W.: Ultrasound instrumentation: Physical principles. *In* Callen, P.W. (Ed.): Ultrasonography in Obstetrics and Gynecology. Philadelphia, W. B. Saunders Co., 1982. Reprinted with permission.)

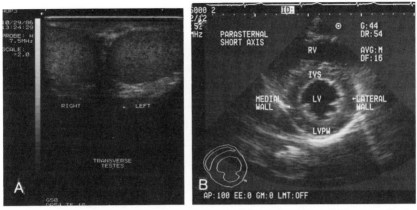

Figure 4.29 Clinical examples of (A) rectangular (bilateral testes) and (B) sector display formats (cardiac left ventricle). (Courtesy of GE Medical Systems.)

Two display formats result from the scanning methods described in the Section 3.4: rectangular and sector (Figs. 4.28 and 4.29). The linear mechanical transducer and the linear switched array produce a rectangular display. The oscillating and rotating mechanical transducers, the oscillating mirror, and the phased array produce a sector display format. In the rectangular format, the scan line density in the display is given in terms of lines per centimeter. This is determined by the lines per frame and the distance in centimeters represented by the width of the rectangular display.

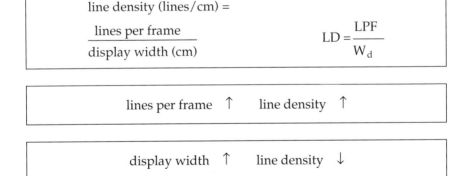

line density (lines/cm) =

$$\frac{\text{lines per frame}}{\text{display width (cm)}} \qquad LD = \frac{LPF}{W_d}$$

lines per frame ↑   line density ↑

display width ↑   line density ↓

For the sector scan format, the line density is determined by the number of lines per frame and the total sector angle (typically 45, 90, or 105 degrees).

$$\text{line density (lines/degree)} = \frac{\text{lines per frame}}{\text{sector angle (degrees)}} \qquad LD = \frac{LPF}{SA}$$

lines per frame ↑   line density ↑

sector angle ↑   line density ↓

For many years diagnostic ultrasound displays used cathode ray storage tubes that could not display various brightnesses. The amplitude of the pulse delivered by the receiver had little effect on the brightness of the spot displayed. The bright spots either were there or were not there. This is referred to as bistable display (on or off). In common use now is gray-scale display, in which several values of brightness may be stored and displayed. These displays produce B scan presentations in which brightness is determined by received reflection amplitude. Higher amplitude reflections may be presented as brighter (white echo) spots or as darker (black echo) spots. In some instruments, either display method may be chosen. White echo is the common method used today.

The scan converter (Section 4.4) is a device that has made stored gray-scale displays possible. It stores the gray-scale image and allows it to be displayed on a television monitor. Gray-scale presentation of reflections preserves some of their dynamic range. Scan converters are capable of storing a greater dynamic range of brightness than the eye can handle. However, photography of displayed images usually limits the dynamic range to less than that of the eye.

M mode display is usually recorded by a strip-chart recorder. B scan freeze-frame displays are usually recorded by photography. B scan real-time displays are recorded on videotape or disc.

For measurement purposes, most displays include range marker dots or calipers, or both. Marker dots are presented as a series of dots in a line with given separation (e.g., 1 cm). Calipers are two pluses (or some other symbol), which can be placed anywhere on the display. The distance between them is calculated by the instrument and read out on the display.

Television monitors are commonly used as the display devices for

Figure 4.30   The television display format has 525 horizontal display scan lines, which are written out in one thirtieth of a second. Half of these (alternate solid lines) are written first, followed by the remaining (dashed) ones. Each of these sets of lines (solid and dashed on this illustration) makes up a "field." Two fields make a frame. Writing the frame in the format of two fields reduces flicker.

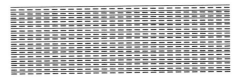

ultrasound imaging instruments. A television monitor is a cathode ray tube in which a particular electron beam scanning format is utilized. The electron beam current is continually changed as the beam is scanned to provide varying brightness of the spot, thus providing gray-scale imaging capability. The television scanning format consists of a left-to-right and top-to-bottom scanning pattern similar to the way in which this page of text is read. The resulting display consists of 525 horizontal display scan lines that produce one frame of a dynamic image (Fig. 4.30). This picture is updated (dynamic imaging) 30 times each second. This compares to motion picture film, in which 24 frames per second are used.

Exercises

4.5.1 The common methods of image presentation are called _____ mode, _____ mode, _____ mode, and _____ scan.

4.5.2 Match the following display modes with the appropriate statements (answers may be used more than once):

a. A mode: _____, _____

b. B mode: _____, _____

c. M mode: _____, _____, _____

d. B scan: _____, _____, _____, _____

1. cross-sectional display
2. dot is deflected by return of a reflection
3. dot is brightened by return of a reflection
4. one axis of recording corresponds to time
5. scan lines move with transducer position and orientation
6. requires the transducer to be moved or scanned to develop the image
7. gives a one-dimensional display

4.5.3 The display device used in each mode is a _____ _____ tube.

4.5.4 The spot on a cathode ray tube may be moved by applying voltage to the _____ plates.

4.5.5 In the A mode, the horizontal position of the vertical deflection is determined by pulse travel _____ and thus by reflector _____.

4.5.6 In the A mode, a vertical deflection nearer the left-hand side of the tube face results from a reflector that is nearer the transducer. True or false?

4.5.7 The _____ mode is used for studying the motion of a reflector.

4.5.8 To position a bright spot on the display in the B mode, the instrument uses the arrival _____ of the reflection and must assume a value for _____ _____ in tissue.

4.5.9 The B scan presents a cross section through the _____ plane.

4.5.10 A display that preserves some of the reflector dynamic range is called a _____ display.

4.5.11 The _____ _____ stores the gray-scale image and allows it to be displayed on a television monitor.

4.5.12 Television monitors produce _____ images per second.
   a. 10
   b. 15
   c. 30
   d. 60
   e. 100

4.5.13 How many horizontal lines are used to produce a picture on a television monitor?
   a. 60
   b. 100
   c. 256
   d. 525
   e. 1024

4.5.14 It takes _____ μs of time to produce a single picture on a television monitor using the television scan format.

4.5.15 It takes _____ μs of time to write one horizontal line of brightness information on a television monitor.

4.5.16 Match the following:
   Real-time transducer   Display
   a. linear mechanical _____   1. rectangular
   b. oscillating _____   2. sector
   c. rotating _____
   d. rotating mirror _____
   e. linear switched
      array _____
   f. linear phased array _____

4.5.17 If the pulse repetition frequency of an instrument is 1 kHz and it displays 25 frames per second, there are _____ lines per frame.

4.5.18 The pulse repetition frequency is _____ Hz if there are 30 frames (40 lines each) per second.

4.5.19 If the instruments have rectangular displays with width representing 10 cm, the line densities for Exercises 4.5.17 and 4.5.18 are _____ and _____ lines/cm, respectively.

4.5.20 If the instruments have sector displays representing 90 degrees, the line densities for Exercises 4.5.17 and 4.5.18 are _____ and _____ lines/degree, respectively.

4.6
Review

Diagnostic ultrasound imaging systems are of the reflection (pulse-echo) type. These use the direction, strength, and arrival time of received reflections to generate a one-dimensional A mode or M mode display or to generate a two-dimensional gray-scale B mode display. Imaging systems consist of a pulser, a transducer, a receiver, a memory, and a display. Receivers amplify, compensate, compress, demodulate, and reject. Compensation equalizes differences in received reflection amplitudes caused by reflector depth. The A mode uses deflection display. The M and B modes use a brightness display. The M mode shows reflector motion in time. The B scan shows a cross section through the scanning plane. Scan converters (memories) store gray-scale image information and permit display on a television monitor. Analog scan converters store echo information as electric charge on a matrix of insulators. Digital scan converters are computer memories that store echo information as numbers in memory elements. Dynamic (real-time) imaging is the rapid sequential display of static ultrasound images resulting in a moving presentation. Such imaging requires rapid, repeatable, sequential scanning of the sound beam through the tissue. This is accomplished by mechanical real-time transducers of various types and by linear switched or phased transducer arrays. Rectangular or sector display formats result from such scanning techniques. Frame rates are typically 10 to 60 per second.

Definitions of terms discussed in this chapter are listed below:

A mode. Mode of operation in which the display records a vertical spot deflection for each pulse delivered from the receiver.

Amplification. Increasing small voltages to larger ones.

Amplifier. A device that accomplishes amplification.

Analog. Related to a procedure or system in which data are represented by continuously variable physical quantities (e.g., electric charge).

B mode. Mode of operation in which the display records a spot brightening for each echo pulse delivered from the receiver.

B scan. A brightness image that represents a cross section of the object through the scanning plane.

Bistable. Having two possible states (e.g., on or off; white or black).

Bistable display. Display in which all recorded spots have the same brightness.

Bit. Binary digit.

Cathode ray tube. A display device that produces an image by scanning an electron beam over a phosphor-coated screen.

Compensation. Equalizing received reflection amplitude differences caused by different attenuations for different reflector depths.

Compression. Decreasing differences between small and large amplitudes.

Contrast resolution. Ability of a gray-scale display to distinguish between echoes of slightly different amplitude or intensity.

Demodulation. Converting voltage pulses from one form to another.

Digital. Related to a procedure or system in which data are represented by discrete units (numerical digits).

Dynamic focusing. Continuously variable received focus that follows the changing position of the transmitted pulse.

Dynamic imaging. Rapid-frame-sequence imaging.

Dynamic range. Ratio (in decibels) of largest power to smallest power that a system can handle or of the largest to the smallest intensity of a group of echoes.

Frame. Display image produced by one complete scan of the sound beam.

Frame rate. Number of frames displayed per unit time.

Gain. Ratio of output to input electric power.

Gray scale. Continuous range of brightnesses between white and black.

Gray-scale display. Display in which several values of spot brightness may be displayed.

M mode. Mode of operation in which the display presents a spot brightening for each pulse delivered from the receiver, producing a two-dimensional recording of reflector position (motion) versus time.

Pixel. Picture element. The unit into which imaging information is divided for storage and display in a digital instrument.

Real-time. Imaging with a real-time display.

Real-time display. A display that continuously images moving structures.

Rejection. Eliminating smaller-amplitude voltage pulses.

Scan converter. A device that stores imaging information in one scanning format and reads it out for display in another.

Scan line. A line produced on a display by moving a spot (produced by an electron beam) across the display face at constant speed.

Scanning. Sweeping a sound beam to produce an image.

Static imaging. Single-frame imaging.

TGC. Time gain compensation (see Compensation).

Variable focusing. Transmit focus with various focal lengths.

Exercises

4.6.1 The reflector information that can be obtained from an M mode display includes
a. distance and motion pattern
b. transducer frequency, reflection coefficient, and distance
c. acoustic impedances, attenuation, and motion pattern
d. none of the above

4.6.2 The compensation (swept gain, and so forth) control serves to
   a. compensate for machine instability in the warm-up time
   b. compensate for attenuation
   c. compensate for transducer aging and the ambient light in the examining area
   d. decrease patient examination time

4.6.3 A gray-scale display shows
   a. gray color on a white background
   b. reflections with one brightness level
   c. a white color on a gray background
   d. a range of reflection amplitudes

4.6.4 The dynamic range of an ultrasound system is defined as
   a. the speed with which ultrasound examination can be performed
   b. the range over which the scanning arm can be manipulated while performing an examination
   c. the ratio of the maximum amplitude to the minimum amplitude or power that can be displayed
   d. the range of pulser voltages applied to the transducer

4.6.5 A digital scan converter is a _____.
   a. compressor
   b. receiver
   c. display
   d. computer memory
   e. none of the above

4.6.6 Place the following in the order in which they are performed in a receiver:
   a. rejection
   b. amplification
   c. smoothing
   d. rectification
   e. compression
   f. compensation

4.6.7 Television displays produce _____ frames per second with _____ lines in each.
   a. 30, 60
   b. 30, 525
   c. 60, 512
   d. 512, 512
   e. 60, 120

4.6.8 In a digital instrument, echo intensity is represented by
   a. positive charge distribution
   b. a number stored in memory

c. electron density of the scan converter writing beam

d. a and c

e. all of the above

4.6.9 If there were no attenuation in tissue, _____ would not be needed.

a. rejection

b. compression

c. demodulation

d. compensation

4.6.10 The television scanning format uses _____ fields per frame so that there are _____ fields presented on the monitor per second.

4.6.11 Which of the following are capable of displaying gray-scale information?

a. storage cathode ray tube

b. television monitor

c. demodulator

d. a and b

e. none of the above

4.6.12 Reflection imaging includes ultrasound generation, propagation and reflection in tissues, and reception of returning _____.

4.6.13 Virtually all the diagnostic ultrasound systems in use today are of the _____ type.

4.6.14 Reflection-type instruments are also called _____ instruments.

4.6.15 Reflection-type instruments look for three things: the _____, _____, and arrival _____ of reflections that occur in tissues.

4.6.16 An analog scan converter stores image information in the form of _____.

a. electric charge

b. digital number

c. resistor temperature

d. impedance

e. none of the above

4.6.17 Imaging systems produce a visual _____ from the electrical _____ received from the transducer.

4.6.18. The transducer is connected to the memory through the _____.

4.6.19. The transducer receives voltages from the _____ in pulse-echo systems.

4.6.20 The _____ receives voltages from the transducer.

4.6.21 Increasing gain generally produces the same effect as
  a. decreasing attenuation
  b. increasing attenuation
  c. increasing compression
  d. increasing rectification
  e. both b and c
4.6.22 Voltage pulses occur at the output of the
  a. pulser
  b. transducer
  c. receiver
  d. display
  e. both a and b
  f. both c and e
4.6.23 Ultrasound pulses from the pulser are applied to the
  a. pulser
  b. transducer
  c. receiver
  d. display
4.6.24 Rectification and smoothing are parts of
  a. amplipression
  b. rejection
  c. a and b
  d. compression
  e. demodulation
4.6.25 If gain is reduced by one half, and if input power is unchanged, the output power is _____ what it was before.
  a. equal to
  b. twice
  c. one half
  d. none of the above
4.6.26 If gain was 30 dB and output power is reduced by one half, the new gain is _____ dB.
  a. 15
  b. 60
  c. 33
  d. 27
  e. none of the above
4.6.27 If four shades of gray are shown on a display, each twice the brightness of the preceding one, the brightest shade is _____ times the brightness of the dimmest shade.
  a. 2
  b. 4
  c. 8

　　　d. 16

　　　e. 32

4.6.28 The dynamic range displayed in Exercise 4.6.27 is _____ dB.

　　　a. 10

　　　b.   9

　　　c.   5

　　　d.   2

　　　e.   0

4.6.29 Gain and attenuation are usually given in

　　　a. dB

　　　b. dB/cm

　　　c. cm

　　　d. cm/3 dB

　　　e. none of the above

4.6.30 Compensation (swept gain) makes up for the fact that reflections from deeper reflectors arrive at the transducer with greater amplitude. True or false?

4.6.31 The modes that show one-dimensional real-time images are the _____ mode and the _____ mode.

4.6.32 The mode that can show two-dimensional real-time images is the _____ mode.

4.6.33 A real-time B mode display may be produced by rapid _____ transducer scanning or by _____ scanning of a transducer array.

4.6.34 Each complete scan of the sound beam produces an image on the display that is called a _____.

4.6.35 The number of lines in each frame is equal to the number of times the transducer is _____ while the frame is produced (while the sound beam is scanned).

4.6.36 In real-time scanning, the pulse repetition frequency is equal to the number of _____ per frame times the _____ rate.

4.6.37 Real-time imaging permits imaging of the motion of moving structures, but it is not as convenient as static B mode imaging for acquiring desired static images. True or false?

4.6.38 In order to correct for attenuation, the TGC must (increase or decrease) _____ the amplification (gain) for increasing depth.

4.6.39 If a higher frequency is used, resolution is (improved or worsened), imaging depth (increases or decreases), and TGC slope must be (increased or decreased)?

4.6.40 Images are typically divided into 512 pixels on each side (512 x 512). This means that an image typically contains how many pixels?

4.6.41 Which type of real-time scanner gives a wide view close to the transducer? Which of the following give(s) a sector format image?
   a. mechanical real-time
   b. linear array
   c. phased array
   d. all of the above

4.6.42 Although dynamic imaging does not require a memory, most real-time scanners have one. It is necessary in order to have _____ _____ capability.

4.6.43 If a real-time scanner produces 1000 pulses per second and 20 frames per second, how many scan lines make up each frame?

Chapter 5

Imaging Artifacts

5.1
Introduction

In imaging, an artifact is anything not properly indicative of the structures imaged. It is caused by some characteristic of the imaging technique. Because some artifacts are useful (e.g., shadowing, enhancement, speed error), imaging can at times be better than direct viewing of the anatomy (if it were possible). This is because some ultrasound imaging artifacts, although errors from an anatomic imaging standpoint, give valuable information on the nature of objects or lesions that might not be apparent with other imaging methods or even direct viewing. In addition to helpful artifacts, there are several that hinder proper interpretation and diagnosis. These must be avoided or properly handled when encountered.

Artifacts in ultrasound imaging[17, 18] occur as structures that are one of the following:

1. not real
2. missing
3. improperly located
4. of improper brightness
5. of improper shape
6. of improper size

Some artifacts are produced by improper equipment operation (e.g., improper transducer location and orientation information sent to the display) or settings (e.g., incorrect receiver compensation settings). Others are inherent in the ultrasound diagnostic method and can occur even with proper equipment and technique.

147

Table 5.1
Ultrasound Imaging
Artifacts
of Acoustic Origin

Resolution Group
  1. Axial resolution
  2. Lateral resolution
  3. Speckle
  4. Section thickness

Propagation Group
  1. Reverberation
  2. Refraction
  3. Multipath
  4. Mirror image
  5. Side lobe
  6. Grating lobe

Attenuation Group
  1. Shadowing
  2. Enhancement
  3. Refraction (edge)
     shadowing
  4. Focal enhancement

Miscellaneous Group
  1. Comet tail
  2. Ring-down
  3. Speed error
  4. Range ambiguity

From Kremkau, F.W., and Taylor, K.J.: Artifacts in ultrasound imaging. J. Ultrasound Med., 5:227–237, 1986. Reprinted with permission.

Artifacts that occur in ultrasound imaging are listed in Table 5.1, grouped as they are considered in this chapter.

The assumptions in the design of ultrasound imaging instruments are that sound travels in straight lines, that echoes originate only from objects located on the transducer axis, that the amplitude or intensity of returning echoes is related to the reflecting or scattering properties of distant objects, and that the distance to reflecting or scattering objects is proportional to the round trip travel time (13 µs per centimeter of depth).

In this chapter we consider the following questions: What causes ultrasound images to appear incorrectly? How can specific artifacts be recognized? How can they be properly handled in order to avoid the pitfalls and misdiagnosis that they can cause? The following terms are discussed in this chapter:

enhancement
multipath
multiple reflections

reverberation
shadowing

5.2
Resolution

Lateral and axial resolution limitations are artifactual in nature because a failure to resolve means a loss of detail and two adjacent structures may be visualized as one. Resolution was discussed in Section 3.5
in terms of separation of two reflectors (see Figs. 3.20 and 3.21). If separation is not sufficient, two reflectors are seen as one (missing-reflector
artifact). Resolution also increases the apparent size of a reflector on a
display (Fig. 5.1). The minimum displayed lateral and axial dimensions
will be the beam diameter and one half the spatial pulse length, respectively (Fig. 5.2). Apparent image resolution can be deceiving. This is not
directly related to tissue scattering properties (texture) but is a result of
interference effects of the scattered sound from the distribution of scatterers in the tissue. This phenomenon is called acoustic speckle (see Section 2.5) (Fig. 5.3).

The beam width perpendicular to the scan plane results in section
thickness artifacts—for example, the appearance of false debris in echo-
free areas (Fig. 5.4) and the presentation of cystic objects as solid (e.g.,
gallbladder). This is because the interrogating beam has finite thickness
as it scans through the patient. Echoes are received that originate not
only from the center of the beam but also from the edges.

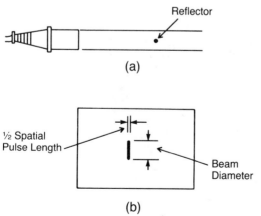

(a)

(b)

Figure 5.1. A tiny reflector (a) is displayed (b) with the axial dimension equal to one-half
the spatial pulse length and the lateral dimension equal to the beam diameter. The image is
produced by scanning the transducer from top to bottom in (a).

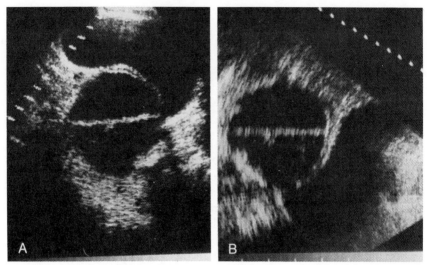

Figure 5.2. Dermoid cyst in the female pelvis. The boundary between lipid and non-lipid regions is presented well axially in (a). In (b), the same boundary appears thicker when imaged laterally with the patient erect. (From Kremkau, F.W., and Taylor, K.J.: Artifacts in ultrasound imaging. J. Ultrasound Med., 5: 227, 1986. Reprinted with permission.)

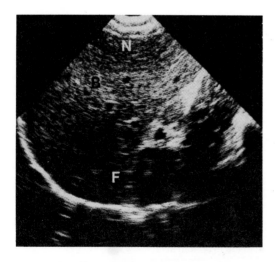

Figure 5.3. Sagittal scan of a normal liver. Lateral resolution is degraded in the far zone (F). Focal banding (B) is seen in the focal region. Apparent resolution in the near zone (N) is partially a result of acoustic speckle. (From Kremkau, F.W., and Taylor, K.J.: Artifacts in ultrasound imaging. J. Ultrasound Med., 5:227, 1986. Reprinted with permission.)

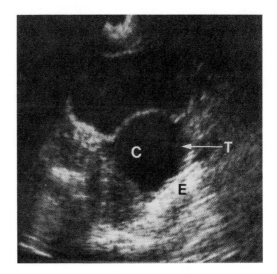

Figure 5.4. A pelvic cyst (C) showing internal section-thickness artifact (T) and distal enhancement (E). (From Kremkau, F.W., and Taylor, K.J.: Artifacts in ultrasound imaging. J. Ultrasound Med., 5:227, 1986. Reprinted with permission.)

5.3
Propagation

If two or more reflectors are encountered in the sound path, multiple reflections (reverberations) will occur. These may be sufficiently strong to be detected by the instrument and to cause confusion on the display. The process by which they are produced is shown in Figure 5.5. This results in placement on the image of reflectors that are not real. They will be placed behind the second real reflector at separation intervals equal to the separation between the first and second real reflectors (Figs. 5.6 to 5.8). Each subsequent reflection is weaker than prior ones, but this will be at least partially compensated for by the compensation function of the receiver.

Refraction (Section 2.5) can cause a reflector to be improperly positioned on the display (Figs. 5.9 to 5.10). A similar occurrence can be caused by reflections from side lobes (Section 3.3) or grating lobes (Section 3.4) (Figs. 5.11 to 5.13).

The term *multipath* describes the situation in which the paths to and from a reflector are different (Fig. 5.14). Multipath results in improper reflector image positioning (increased range).

In a mirror image artifact objects that are present on one side of a strong reflector are presented on the other side as well (Fig. 5.15). This commonly occurs around the diaphragm (Figs. 5.16 and 5.17).

First   Second
Reflector   Reflector

(a)

(b)

(c)

(d)

(e)

(f)

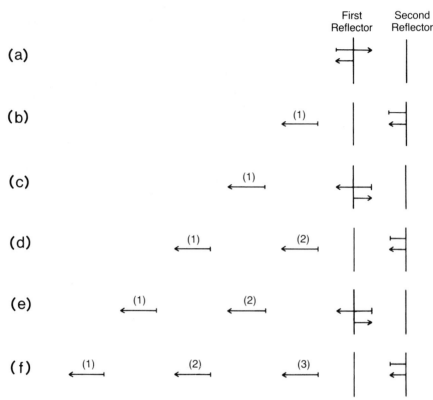

Figure 5.5. The generation of multiple reflections (reverberations). (a) An ultrasound pulse has come from the left, has encountered the first reflector, and has been partially reflected and partially transmitted. (b) Reflection and transmission at the first reflector are complete. Reflection at the second reflector is occurring. (c) Reflection at the second reflector is complete. Partial transmission (from right to left this time) and partial reflection are again occurring at the first reflector. (d) The reflections from the first (1) and second (2) reflectors are traveling to the left toward the sound source. A second reflection (repeat of [b]) is occurring at the second reflector. (e) Partial transmission and reflection are again occurring at the first reflector. (f) Three reflections are now traveling to the left: (1) is the reflection from the first reflector; (2) is the reflection from the second reflector; (3) is the reflection from the second reflector, reflected from the back side of the first reflector (c) and reflected again from the second reflector (d). A fourth reflection is being generated at the second reflector (f). Action proceeds from top to bottom in the figure. The first reflector is sometimes the transducer face.

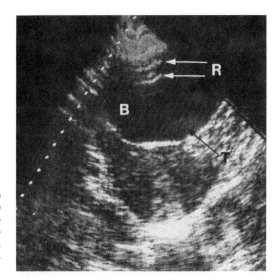

Figure 5.6. Reverberation (R) and section-thickness artifact (T) in the bladder (B). (From Kremkau, F.W., and Taylor, K.J.: Artifacts in ultrasound imaging. J. Ultrasound Med., 5:227, 1986. Reprinted with permission.)

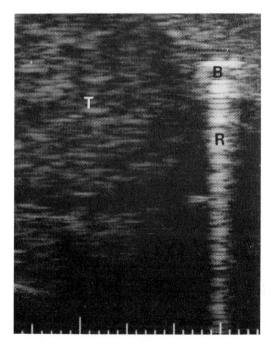

Figure 5.7. Short-range reverberation (R) from an air gun BB (B) adjacent to the testicle (T). (From Kremkau, F.W., and Taylor, K.J.: Artifacts in ultrasound imaging. J. Ultrasound Med., 5:227, 1986. Reprinted with permission.)

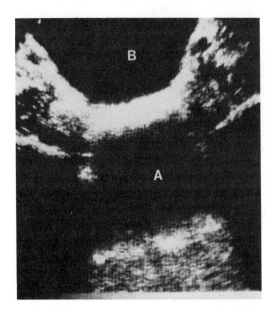

Figure 5.8. Long-range reverberation causes bladder (B) to be imaged a second time (A). (From Kremkau, F.W., and Taylor, K.J.: Artifacts in ultrasound imaging. J. Ultrasound Med., 5:227, 1986. Reprinted with permission.)

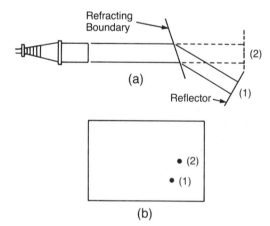

Figure 5.9. Improper positioning of the reflector on the display (b) because of refraction (a). The system thinks the reflector is at position 2 because that is the direction in which the transducer is pointing. The reflector is actually at position 1.

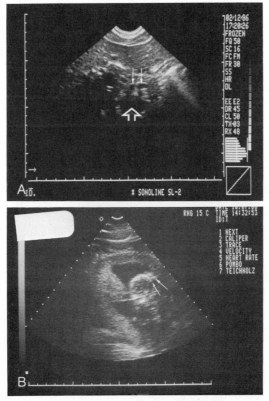

Figure 5.10. (a) Refraction (probably through the rectus abdominis muscle) has widened the aorta (open arrow) and produced a double image of the celiac trunk (arrows). (b) Refraction has produced a double image of a fetal skull (arrows).

Figure 5.11. A side lobe or grating lobe can produce and receive a reflection from a "side view." This will be placed on the display at the proper distance from the transducer but in the wrong location (direction). This is because the instrument assumes that echoes originate from points along the transducer axis (the direction in which it is pointing). The instrument thinks that the reflector is at position 2 because that is the direction in which the transducer is pointing. The reflector is actually in position 1.

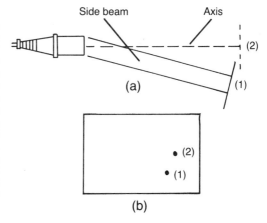

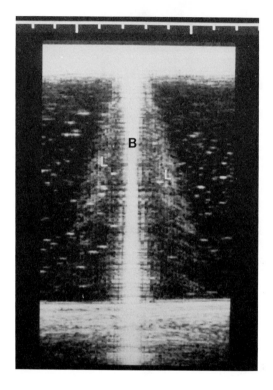

Figure 5.12. Primary beam (B) and side lobes (L) from a linear-array transducer.

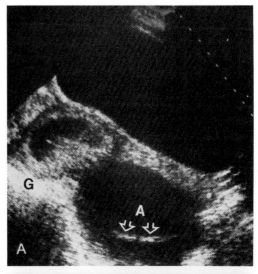

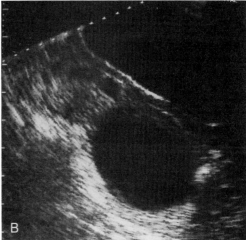

Figure 5.13. (a) Side lobe artifact (A) appears in a scan of a corpus luteal cyst but not in other scans of the same cyst. The reflector generating this artifact is likely bowel gas (G). (b) Another scan which does not pass through the location of the gas does not have the artifact present in the cyst. [(a) From Kremkau, F.W., and Taylor, K.J.: Artifacts in ultrasound imaging. J. Ultrasound Med., 5:227, 1986. Reprinted with permission.]

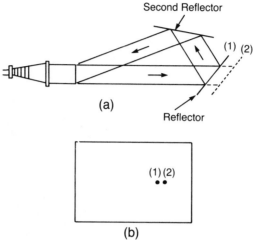

Figure 5.14. Improper positioning of the reflector on the display (b) because of multipath (a). The instrument thinks that the reflector is at position 2 because of the increased round-trip travel time required for a longer return path. The reflector is actually at position 1.

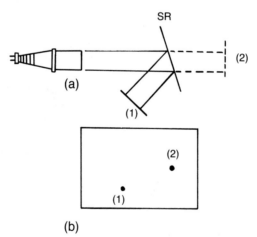

Figure 5.15. The mirror-image artifact occurs around strong reflectors (SR). The reflector that is located in position 1 is imaged in position 2 because that is the direction in which the transducer is pointing.

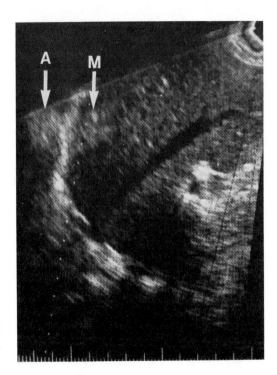

Figure 5.16. Anechoic mass (M) in the liver is also artifactually represented (A) superior to the diaphragm. (From Kremkau, F.W., and Taylor, K.J.: Artifacts in ultrasound imaging. J. Ultrasound Med., 5:227, 1986. Reprinted with permission.)

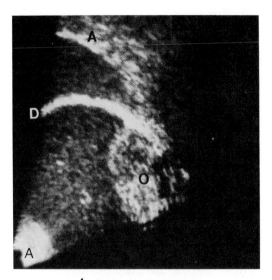

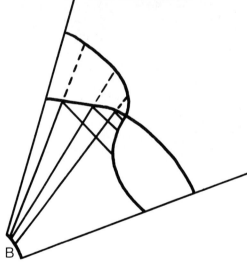

Figure 5.17. (a) An unusual presentation (A) of mirror-image artifact around the diaphragm (D). The shape of the artifact (A) is not the same as that of the object (O) (probably bowel). The explanation of this result is shown in (b). (From Kremkau, F.W., and Taylor, K.J.: Artifacts in ultrasound imaging. J. Ultrasound Med., 5:227, 1986. Reprinted with permission.)

5.4
Attenuation

Shadowing is the reduction in reflection amplitude from reflectors that lie behind a strongly reflecting (Fig. 5.18) or attenuating (Fig. 5.19) structure. Enhancement is the increase in reflection amplitude from reflectors that lie behind a weakly attenuating structure (Figs. 5.18 and 5.20). Shadowing and enhancement result in reflectors being placed on the image with amplitudes that are too low and too high, respectively. Brightening of echoes can also be due to the increased intensity in the focal region of a beam. This is called focal enhancement or focal banding (Fig. 5.3). Shadowing and enhancement can also occur behind the edges of objects that are not necessarily strong or weak attenuators (Figs. 5.21 and 5.22). In this case the cause is the focusing or defocusing action of a refracting curved surface (Fig. 5.23). This increases or decreases the intensity of the beam beyond the surface, causing echoes to be strengthened or weakened. Shadowing and enhancement are useful artifacts for determining the nature of masses.

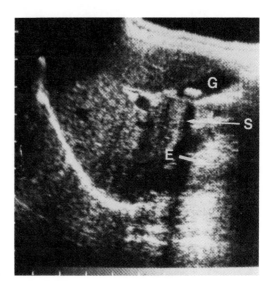

Figure 5.18. Shadowing (S) from a gallstone (G) and enhancement (E) from the gallbladder. (From Kremkau, F.W., and Taylor, K.J.: Artifacts in ultrasound imaging. J. Ultrasound Med., 5:227, 1986. Reprinted with permission.)

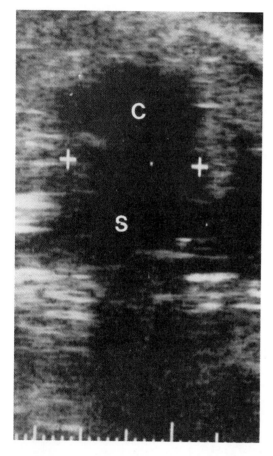

Figure 5.19. Anechoic breast carcinoma (C) with distal shadowing (S). (From Kremkau, F.W., and Taylor, K.J.: Artifacts in ultrasound imaging. J. Ultrasound Med., 5:227, 1986. Reprinted with permission.)

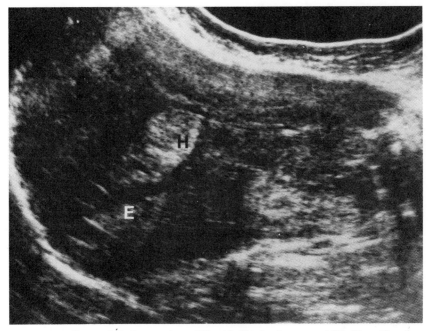

Figure 5.20. Hyperechoic hemangioma (H) with distal enhancement (E). (From Kremkau, F.W., and Taylor, K.J.: Artifacts in ultrasound imaging. J. Ultrasound Med., 5:227, 1986. Reprinted with permission.)

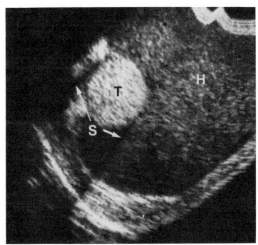

Figure 5.21. Scattering from particles in hematocele (H) simulates a solid mass surrounding the testicle (T). Shadowing from the testicle (or enhancement from hematocele) indicates the cystic nature of this collection. (From Kremkau, F.W., and Taylor, K.J.: Artifacts in ultrasound imaging. J. Ultrasound Med., 5:227, 1986. Reprinted with permission.)

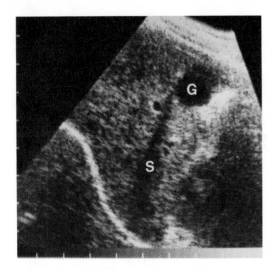

Figure 5.22. Edge shadowing (S) from the gallbladder (G). (From Kremkau, F.W., and Taylor, K.J.: Artifacts in ultrasound imaging. J. Ultrasound Med., 5:227, 1986. Reprinted with permission.)

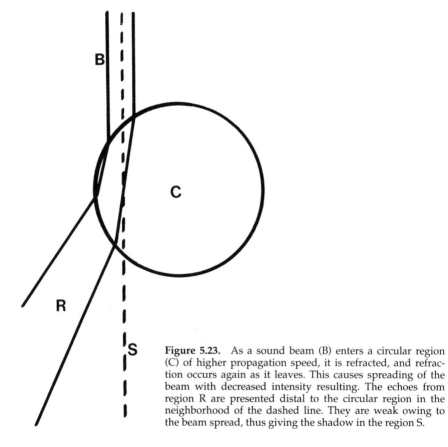

Figure 5.23. As a sound beam (B) enters a circular region (C) of higher propagation speed, it is refracted, and refraction occurs again as it leaves. This causes spreading of the beam with decreased intensity resulting. The echoes from region R are presented distal to the circular region in the neighborhood of the dashed line. They are weak owing to the beam spread, thus giving the shadow in the region S.

5.5
Miscellaneous

Propagation speed error occurs when the assumed value for propagation speed in the range equation (Section 2.5) is incorrect. For diagnostic instruments a speed of 1.54 mm/μs is assumed. If the propagation speed that exists over a path traveled is greater than 1.54 mm/μs, the calculated distance to the reflector is too small, and the display will place the reflector too close to the transducer (Fig. 5.24). If the actual speed is less than 1.54 mm/μs, the reflector will be displayed too far from the transducer (Fig. 5.25). Refraction and propagation speed error can also cause a structure to be displayed with incorrect shape (Fig. 5.25).

In all of the operating modes discussed in Chapter 4, it is assumed that for each pulse, all reflections are received before the next pulse is sent out. If this were not the case, ambiguity could result (Fig. 5.26). The maximum depth to be imaged unambiguously by an instrument determines its maximum pulse repetition frequency. The relationship between the two is:

$$\text{maximum depth (cm)} = \frac{77}{\text{pulse repetition frequency (kHz)}} \qquad d_m = \frac{77}{\text{PRF}}$$

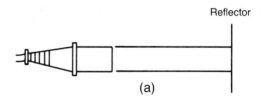

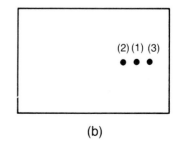

(a)

(b)

Figure 5.24. Reflector position on the display (b) depends on the propagation speed over the traveled path (a). The reflector is actually in position 1. If the actual propagation speed is less than that assumed, the reflector will appear in position 3. If the actual speed is more than that assumed, the reflector will appear in position 2.

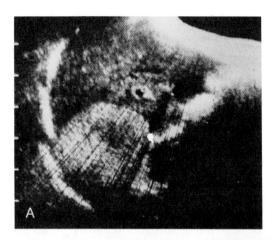

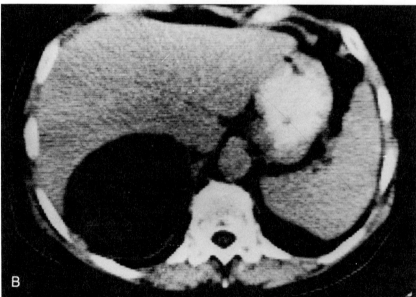

Figure 5.25. (a) Adrenal myelolipoma with 11-cm axial dimension on ultrasound scan. The distal diaphragm is displaced 2 cm. (b) CT image of this 9-cm tumor. [(a) From Richman, T.S., Taylor, K.J., Kremkau, F.W.: Propagation speed artifact in a fatty tumor (myelolipoma): Significance for tissue differential diagnosis. J. Ultrasound Med., 2: 45, 1983. Reprinted with permission.]

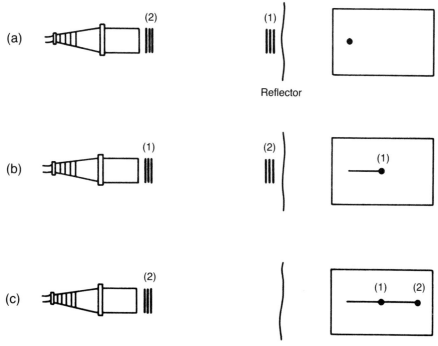

Figure 5.26. Ambiguity caused by sending out a pulse before a reflection from the previous pulse is received. (a) A pulse (2) is sent out just as a previous pulse (1) is reflected. (b) The spot begins to move across the display. The first reflection arrives at the transducer when the second pulse reflects. (c) The second reflection arrives at the transducer, putting a bright spot (2) on the display at the position corresponding to the reflector. The spot (1) in the center of the display resulting from the arrival of the earlier pulse indicates a reflector at a location where there is none.

> pulse repetition frequency ↑   maximum depth ↓

In dynamic imaging, the pulse repetition frequency, the number of lines per frame, and the number of frames per second (frame rate) are related to one another (Section 4.5):

> pulse repetition frequency (Hz) = lines per frame x frame rate
> PRF = LPF x FR

> lines per frame ↑   pulse repetition frequency ↑

> frame rate ↑   pulse repetition frequency ↑

The relationship of lines per frame, frame rate, and maximum imaging depth in soft tissue is:

> maximum depth (cm) x lines per frame x frame rate = 77,000
> d_m x LPF x FR = 77,000

> lines per frame ↑   maximum depth ↓

> frame rate ↑   maximum depth ↓

For example, if the maximum imaging depth desired is 20 cm and the frame rate is 20 frames per second, approximately 200 lines per frame maximum will be permitted to avoid ambiguity. If imaging at a greater depth is desired, either the frame rate or the lines per frame will have to be reduced. The 77,000 comes from one half the propagation speed in centimeters per second. Table 5.2 gives various values for pulse repetition frequency and maximum unambiguous imaging depth. Table 5.3 lists values of lines per frame, frame rate, and depth for dynamic imaging. When imaging with higher frequencies, greater attenuation limits imaging depth, thus allowing more lines per frame or higher frame rate, or both.

An example of a particularly well localized "enhancement" phenomenon, which has been termed comet-tail artifact, is shown in Figure 5.27. It appears to be a series of closely spaced discrete echoes similar to the short-range reverberation in Figure 5.7. The examples in Figure 5.28 appear to be fundamentally different from this. Discrete echoes cannot be identified because they are too close together or, rather, a continuous emission of sound from the origin may be occurring. The mechanism for such a continuous effect (termed ring-down artifact) is not well understood, but it may be caused by a resonance phenomenon associated with gas bubbles.

In addition to the individual artifacts discussed in this chapter, sometimes one artifact can mimic another, and sometimes more than one

Table 5.2
Pulse Repetition Frequency (PRF)
and Maximum Unambiguous Depth
to Avoid Range Ambiguity

PRF (kHz)	Depth (cm)
7.7	10
3.8	20
2.6	30
1.0	77
2.0	38
3.0	26

can combine to produce a complicated artifactual image that can be very confusing and misleading. Figure 5.29 is an example of the former. Enhancement appears to occur where unexpected. The liver and an anechoic mass within or adjacent to the diaphragm are shown. Enhancement appears to be present in the lung. On closer inspection it is seen that this apparent enhanced transmission is, rather, presentation of two reverberations from within the anechoic mass. The strong echo from the air boundary superior to the diaphragm appears distal to the mass (as it should). This boundary is then imaged two more times (superior to the diaphragm) as a result of reverberation.

In conclusion, an interesting and sobering case is presented. Figure 5.30a shows an image of a hemorrhagic corpus luteal cyst. Figure 5.30b shows a similar-appearing pelvic collection in a patient in whom we were searching for an abscess. This pelvic collection is completely artifactual! Another view with the distended urinary bladder completely filling the pelvis (the patient had had a hysterectomy) is shown in Figure 5.30c. The coccyx produced a distal shadow. Reverberation in the bladder images the coccyx a second time. Distal filling (in Fig. 5.30b) occurs this

Table 5.3
Lines per Frame (LPF), Frames per Second (Frame rate: FR), and Maximum Depth to Avoid Dynamic Imaging Range Ambiguity*

LPF	FR	Depth (cm)
1540	10	5
513	30	5
308	50	5
770	10	10
257	30	10
154	50	10
385	10	20
128	30	20
77	50	20

*LPF x FR = pulse repetition frequency (PRF in Table 5.2)

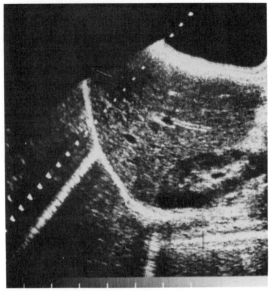

Figure 5.27.   Comet-tail from the diaphragm. (From Kremkau, F.W., and Taylor, K.J.: Artifacts in ultrasound imaging. J. Ultrasound Med., 5:227, 1986. Reprinted with permission.)

time because time gain compensation has overincreased the gain (relatively low attenuation in the urine). This deceiving image resulted from the combination of three artifacts—shadowing, reverberation, and enhancement. The artifactual mass is totally located outside the patient, whose outer margin is indicated by the arrows in Figure 5.30c.

5.6
Review

Axial resolution is determined by spatial pulse length. Lateral resolution is determined by beam width. Apparent resolution close to the transducer is not directly related to tissue texture but is a result of interference effects from a distribution of scatterers in the tissue. The beam width perpendicular to the scan plane results in slice thickness artifacts. Reverberation produces a set of equally spaced artifactual echoes distal to the real reflector. In a mirror image artifact objects that are present on one side of a strong reflector are presented on the other side as well. Enhancement results from low attenuation objects in the sound path. Propagation speed error and refraction can cause objects to be displayed improperly in location or size, or both. Refraction can also cause edge shadowing or enhancement.

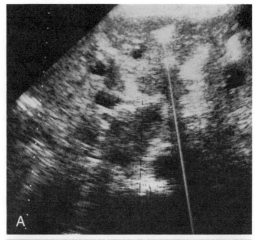

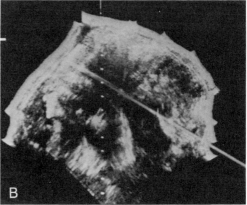

Figure 5.28. Ring-down from (a) air in the bile duct and (b) bowel. [(a) From Kremkau, F.W., and Taylor, K.J.: Artifacts in ultrasound imaging. J. Ultrasound Med., 5:227, 1986. Reprinted with permission.]

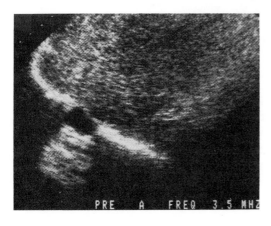

Figure 5.29. A case of reverberation mimicking enhancement. An anechoic mass is located at the diaphragm. The apparent enhanced transmission distal to the mass (into the lung) is a result of two reverberations within the anechoic mass. (From Kremkau, F.W., and Taylor, K.J.: Artifacts in ultrasound imaging. J. Ultrasound Med., 5:227, 1986. Reprinted with permission.)

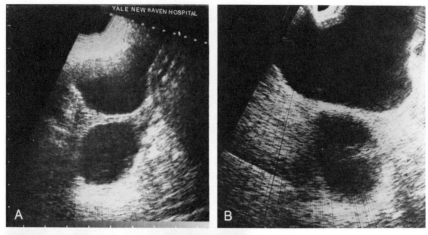

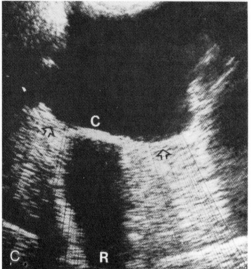

Figure 5.30. (a) A hemorrhagic corpus-luteal cyst. (b) Apparent pelvic collection. (c) A second view of the collection shown in (b) that indicates its artifactual nature. The distended urinary bladder compresses the empty rectum and completely fills the pelvis (the patient had had a hysterectomy). The outer margin of the patient (determined by measurement) is indicated by the arrows. The coccyx (C) produces a distal shadow. Reverberation (R), i.e., a second image of the coccyx, and enhancement from increased gain (TGC) on the second round-trip fill in the shadow posteriorly. The combination of shadowing, reverberation, and enhancement produces the convincing but totally artifactual mass seen in (b). ([b] and [c] from Kremkau, F.W., and Taylor, K.J.: Artifacts in ultrasound imaging. J. Ultrasound Med., 5:227, 1986. Reprinted with permission.)

In this chapter we have discussed 18 ultrasound imaging artifacts of acoustic origin. They are listed in Table 5.4 according to the ways in which they are manifested. Explanations of how these artifacts occur are listed in Table 5.5. In some cases, artifact names are identical to their causes.

Some artifacts are useful in interpretation and diagnosis (e.g., shadowing and enhancement), whereas some can cause confusion and

Table 5.4
Artifacts Listed by Manifestation

Added Objects	Missing Objects	Incorrect Object Brightness
Speckle	Resolution	Shadowing
Section thickness		Enhancement
Reverberation		
Mirror image		
Comet-tail		
Ring-down		

Incorrect Object Location	Incorrect Object Size	Incorrect Object Shape
Refraction	Resolution	Resolution
Multipath	Refraction	Refraction
Side lobe	Speed error	Speed error
Grating lobe		
Speed error		
Range ambiguity		

From Kremkau, F.W., and Taylor, K.J.: Artifacts in ultrasound imaging. J. Ultrasound Med., 5:227–237, 1986. Reprinted with permission.

error (e.g., section thickness and reverberation). A proper understanding of artifacts and how to deal with them when encountered enables sonographers and sonologists to use them in diagnosis while avoiding the pitfalls which they can cause.

Table 5.5
Artifacts and Their Causes

Artifact	Cause
Axial resolution	Pulse length
Lateral resolution	Pulse width
Speckle	Interference
Section thickness	Pulse width
Reverberation	Reflection
Refraction	Refraction
Multipath	Reflection
Mirror image	Reflection
Side lobe	Side lobe
Grating lobe	Grating lobe
Shadowing	Attenuation
Enhancement	Attenuation (low)
Refraction shadowing	Refraction
Focal enhancement	Focusing
Comet-tail	Reverberation
Ring-down	Resonance
Speed error	Speed error
Range ambiguity	High pulse repetition frequency

From Kremkau, F.W., and Taylor, K.J.: Artifacts in ultrasound imaging. J. Ultrasound Med., 5:227–237, 1986. Reprinted with permission.

Definitions of terms discussed in this chapter are listed below:

Enhancement. Increase in reflection amplitude from reflectors that lie behind a weakly attenuating structure.

Multipath. Paths to and from a reflector are not the same.

Multiple reflections. Several reflections produced by a pulse encountering a pair of reflectors.

Reverberation. Multiple reflections.

Shadowing. Reduction in reflection amplitude from reflectors that lie behind a strongly reflecting or attenuating structure.

Exercises

5.6.1 The maximum pulse repetition frequency that will unambiguously image to a maximum depth of 15 cm is _____ kHz.

5.6.2 The maximum depth for unambiguous imaging with an instrument having a pulse repetition frequency of 1 kHz is _____ cm.

5.6.3 If the propagation speed in a soft tissue path is 1.60 mm/μs, a diagnostic instrument assumes a propagation speed too _____ and will show reflectors too _____ the transducer.
   a. high, close to
   b. high, far from
   c. low, close to
   d. low, far from

5.6.4 Multipath can occur with only one reflector. True or false?

5.6.5 The minimum displayed axial dimension of a reflector is equal to
   a. beam diameter
   b. ½ x beam diameter
   c. 2 x beam diameter
   d. spatial pulse length
   e. ½ x spatial pulse length
   f. 2 x spatial pulse length

5.6.6 The minimum displayed lateral dimension of a reflector is approximately equal to
   a. beam diameter
   b. ½ x beam diameter

    c. 2 x beam diameter

    d. spatial pulse length

    e. ½ x spatial pulse length

    f. 2 x spatial pulse length

5.6.7 The fine texture in the region near the transducer indicates the extremely excellent resolution that actually exists in that region. True or false?

5.6.8 The fact that a beam, as it scans through tissue, has some finite width results in the _____ _____ artifact.

5.6.9 Which of the following can cause improper location of objects on a display? (More than one correct answer)

    a. shadowing

    b. enhancement

    c. speed error

    d. mirror image

    e. refraction

    f. side lobe

5.6.10 Refraction can cause shadowing. True or false?

5.6.11 The transducer face is one of the reflectors involved in reverberations in which illustration (Fig. 5.7 or 5.8)?

5.6.12 Match these artifact causes with their results:

    a. reverberation: _____   1. unreal structure displayed

    b. shadowing: _____, _____   2. structure missing on the display

    c. enhancement: _____   3. structure displayed with

    d. curved reflector: _____   improper brightness

    e. oblique reflector: _____,   4. improperly positioned structure

    _____   5. improperly shaped structure

    f. propagation speed error: 6. structure of improper size

    _____, _____

    g. refraction: _____, _____

    h. multipath: _____

    i. resolution: _____, _____

5.6.13 Reverberation results in added reflectors being imaged with equal _____.

5.6.14 In reverberation, subsequent reflections are _____ than previous ones.

5.6.15 Enhancement is caused by a

    a. strongly reflecting structure

    b. weakly attenuating structure

    c. strongly attenuating structure

    d. refracting boundary

    e. propagation speed error

5.6.16 A reflector may be missing from the display because of
   a. reverberation
   b. propagation speed error
   c. enhancement
   d. oblique reflection
   e. Doppler shift
   f. resonance

5.6.17 Shadowing results in decreased reflection amplitudes. True or false?

5.6.18 Propagation speed error results in improper _____ position of a reflector on the display.
   a. lateral
   b. axial

5.6.19 If the maximum depth imaged is 20 cm and the frame rate is 20 frames per second, there can be, at most, _____ lines per frame.

5.6.20 The pulse repetition frequency in Exercise 5.6.19 is _____ kHz.

5.6.21 If there are 200 lines per frame and 25 frames per second, can 20 cm of depth be imaged unambiguously?

5.6.22 Which artifact should be suspected if observing twin gestational sacs when scanning through the rectus abdominis muscle?

Chapter 6

Doppler Instruments

6.1
Introduction

One item of information not used by the instruments described in Chapter 4 is the doppler shift of the received reflections. Doppler instruments respond to moving reflectors or scatterers (usually blood cells in circulation) by detecting doppler shift.[19-21] This information is converted to audible sound and to a visual display. Doppler instruments are of three types:

1. continuous-wave
2. pulsed-wave
3. color-flow

Doppler instrument SPTA intensities[13-16] range from 0.2 to 2000 mW/cm^2.

In this chapter we consider the following questions: How does ultrasound detect and measure flow? In what ways is flow information presented? How is flow detection localized to a specific site in tissue? How is two-dimensional flow determined and presented in real-time? The following terms are discussed in this chapter:

aliasing	doppler shift
autocorrelation	fourier transform
bidirectional	frequency spectrum
color flow	generator gate
cosine	receiver gate
doppler angle	spectral broadening
doppler effect	

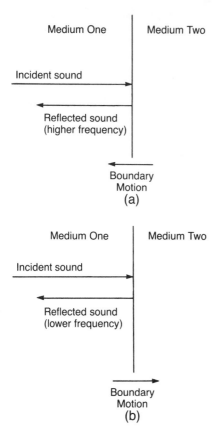

Figure 6.1.   Doppler effect. (a) If the reflector (boundary) moves toward the source, the reflected frequency is higher than the incident frequency. (b) If the reflector moves away from the source, the reflected frequency is lower than the incident frequency.

6.2
Doppler Effect

In Chapter 2 only media boundaries that are stationary with respect to the sound source were considered. If a boundary is moving with respect to the source, the doppler effect will occur. The doppler effect is a change in reflected frequency caused by reflector motion. If the media boundary (reflector) is moving toward the source (Fig. 6.1[a]), the reflected frequency will be higher than the incident frequency. If the reflector is moving away from the source (Fig. 6.1[b]), the reflected frequency will be lower than the incident frequency. The greater the speed of the boundary, the greater will be the difference between incident and reflected frequencies. The incident frequency subtracted from the reflected frequency is called the doppler shift. The doppler equation provides a quantitative relationship between the flow speed and the change in frequency:

doppler shift (MHz) = reflected frequency (MHz) –
incident frequency (MHz) = $f_D = f_r - f_i$

$$\pm \; \frac{2 \times \text{reflector speed (m/s)} \times \text{incident frequency (MHz)}}{\text{propagation speed (m/s)}} \qquad = \pm \frac{2\,S_r\,f_i}{c}$$

reflector speed $\uparrow$ shift $\uparrow$

incident frequency $\uparrow$ shift $\uparrow$

The plus sign is used when the reflector is moving toward the source and the minus sign is used when the reflector is moving away from the source. The doppler shift equation should have the sum of propagation speed and reflector speed in the denominator. However, the use of propagation speed alone is an acceptable approximation because physiologic speeds are small compared with sound speed. If the direction of the incident sound is not parallel to the direction of the boundary motion (Fig. 6.2), the right side of the equation must be multiplied by the cosine (cos) (Appendix C) of the angle between these directions (the doppler angle). Tables 6.1 and 6.2 list doppler frequency shifts for several reflector or scatterer speeds. Tables 6.2 and 6.3 give examples of the effect

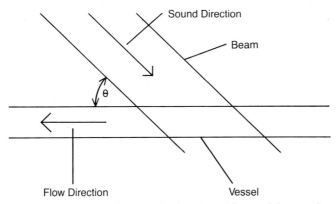

Figure 6.2. Angle θ is the angle between the direction of flow and the sound propagation direction. (From Kremkau, F.W., Technical considerations, equipment, and physics of duplex sonography. *In* Grant, E.G., and White, E.M.: Duplex Sonography. New York, Springer-Verlag, 1988. Reprinted with permission.)

Table 6.1
Doppler Frequency Shifts for Various Scatterer Speeds
Toward the Sound Source*

Incident Frequency (MHz)	Scatterer Speed (c/ms)	Reflected Frequency (MHz)	Doppler Shift (kHz)
2	50	2.0013	1.3
5	50	5.0032	3.2
10	50	10.0065	6.5
2	200	2.0052	5.2
5	200	5.013	13.0
10	200	10.026	26.0

*Motion away from the source would yield negative doppler shifts.

Table 6.2
Doppler Frequency Shifts (f_D) for Various
Frequencies (f), Reflector Speeds (v), and
Angles (θ)*

f (MHz)	v (cm/s)	θ (degrees)	f_D (kHz)
2.5	50	0	1.6
5.0	50	0	3.2
7.5	50	0	4.9
2.5	100	0	3.2
5.0	100	0	6.5
7.5	100	0	9.7
2.5	150	0	4.9
5.0	150	0	9.7
7.5	150	0	14.6
5.0	50	30	2.8
5.0	50	60	1.6
5.0	50	90	0.0
5.0	100	30	5.6
5.0	100	60	3.2
5.0	100	90	0.0
5.0	150	30	8.5
5.0	150	60	4.9
5.0	150	90	0.0
4.0	50	0	2.6
4.0	100	0	5.2
4.0	200	0	10.4
4.0	100	30	4.5
4.0	100	60	2.6
4.0	100	90	0.0
2.0	100	0	2.6
8.0	100	0	10.4

*Flow is toward the transducer (flow away would yield negative doppler shifts). (From Kremkau, F.W.: Technical considerations, equipment, and physics of duplex sonography. *In* Grant E.G., and White, E.M.: Duplex Sonography. New York, Springer-Verlag, 1988. Reprinted with permission.)

Table 6.3
Doppler Frequency Shifts for Various Angles and Scatterer Speeds Toward the Sound Source of Frequency 5 MHz

Scatterer Speed (cm/s)	Angle (°)	Doppler Shift (kHz)
100	0	6.5
100	30	5.6
100	60	3.2
100	90	0.0
300	0	19.0
300	30	17.0
300	60	9.7
300	90	0.0

of angle on doppler shift. Tables 6.2 and 6.3 indicate that for a 90° doppler angle, the doppler shift is zero. In practice there is some doppler shift observed even at a 90° angle because beams are not cylindrical in shape (Fig. 3.8). Thus, even when the beam axis (center line) is perpendicular to the flow, portions of the beam encounter the flow at other (nonperpendicular) angles. An instrument designed to measure the difference between the incident and reflected frequencies can yield information on reflector motion. The moving reflector could be a tissue boundary (e.g., a blood vessel wall or fetal heart) or a cell in suspension (e.g., blood cells in circulation). Commonly used frequencies are in the 2 to 10 MHz range.

The doppler instrument receiver detects and calculates the doppler shift. To get flow speed from that, the angle must be known as well as the speed of sound and the operating frequency, as seen in the following rearranged form of the doppler equation:

$$\text{reflector speed} = \frac{\pm \text{ doppler shift} \times \text{ propagation speed}}{2 \times \text{ incident frequency} \times \cos\theta} \quad S_r = \frac{\pm f_D c}{2 f_i \cos\theta}$$

When the speed of sound (1.54 mm/μs) is inserted, we get:

$$S_r(\text{cm/s}) = \frac{77 f_D(\text{kHz})}{f_i(\text{MHz})\cos\theta}$$

The optimum angle range for most studies is approximately 30 to 60 degrees. For greater angles, the doppler shift becomes too small (except for extremely high flow speeds), and for smaller angles refraction and critical-angle effects inhibit successful signal acquisition.

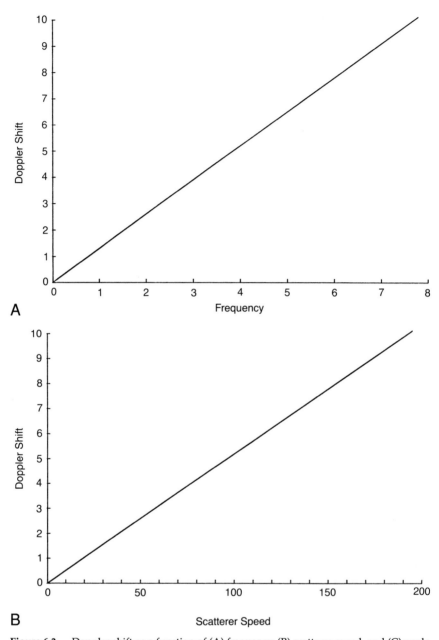

Figure 6.3. Doppler shift as a function of (A) frequency, (B) scatterer speed, and (C) angle as determined by the doppler shift equation. (From Kremkau, F.W.: Seeing and hearing blood flow noninvasively using the doppler shift. Diagn. Imaging, 7:131, 1985. Reprinted with permission.)

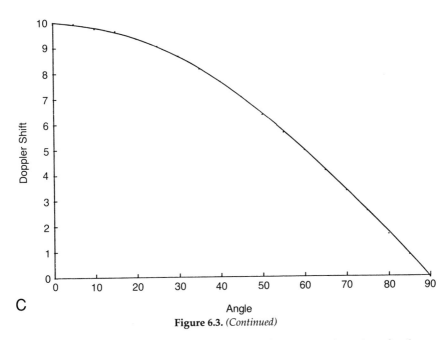

C

Angle

Figure 6.3. *(Continued)*

The fact that the cosine is a rapidly decreasing function for large angles (Table C.1, Appendix C) means that errors in angle measurement are more serious when large angles are involved than they are for small angles. For example, a 10-degree error in angle measurement at a true angle of zero degrees gives a 2 per cent error (cosines of 0 and 10-degree angles are 1.00 and 0.98, respectively), whereas a 10-degree error at 70 degrees yields a 50 per cent error (cosines of 70 and 80 degrees are 0.34 and 0.17, respectively).

The dependence of doppler shift on operating (incident) frequency, scatterer (flow) speed, and doppler angle is shown in Figure 6.3.

Exercises

6.2.1 The doppler effect is a change in reflected _____ caused by reflector _____.

6.2.2 If the reflector is moving toward the source, the reflected frequency is _____ than the incident frequency.

6.2.3 If the reflector is moving away from the source, the reflected frequency is _____ than the incident frequency.

6.2.4 If the reflector is stationary with respect to the source, the reflected frequency is _____ _____ the incident frequency.

6.2.5 Measurement of doppler shift yields information about reflector
_____.

6.2.6 If the incident frequency is 1 MHz, the propagation speed is 1600 m/s, and the reflector speed is 16 m/s toward the source, the doppler shift is _____ MHz and the reflected frequency is _____ MHz.

6.2.7 If 2-MHz ultrasound is reflected from a soft tissue boundary moving at 10 m/s toward the source, the doppler shift is _____ MHz.

6.2.8 If 2-MHz ultrasound is reflected from a soft tissue boundary moving at 10 m/s away from the source, the doppler shift is _____ MHz.

6.2.9 Doppler shift is the difference between _____ and _____ frequencies.

6.2.10 When incident sound direction and reflector motion are not parallel, calculation of the reflected frequency involves the _____ of the angle between these directions.

6.2.11 If the angle between incident sound direction and reflector motion is 60 degrees, the doppler shift and reflected frequency in Exercise 6.2.6 are _____ MHz and _____ MHz.

6.2.12 If the angle between incident sound direction and reflector motion is 90 degrees, the cosine of the angle is _____ and the reflected frequency in Exercise 6.2.6 is _____ MHz.

6.2.13 A policeman in a (doppler) radar-equipped patrol car detects the speed of an automobile to be 55 mph. If the angle between the radar beam and the direction of the automobile is 60 degrees, the actual speed of the automobile is _____ mph.

6.3
Continuous-Wave Instruments

Ultrasound doppler instruments must provide continuous or pulsed voltages to the transducer and convert voltages received from the transducer to audible or visual information corresponding to reflector or scatterer motion. If an instrument can distinguish between positive and negative doppler shifts, it is said to be bidirectional. Continuous-wave doppler instruments consist of a continuous-wave voltage generator and a receiver that converts the change in frequency (doppler shift) resulting from reflector or scatterer motion to an audible sound or to an image corresponding to motion of the objects.

A diagram of the components of a continuous-wave doppler system is given in Figure 6.4. The voltage generator produces continuous voltage of frequency 2 to 10 MHz, which is applied to the source transducer. The ultrasound frequency is determined by the voltage generator. It is set to equal the operating frequency of the transducer (Section 3.2). In the transducer assembly there is a separate receiving transducer that produces a voltage with a frequency equal to the frequency of the reflected ultrasound. If there is reflector motion, the reflected ultrasound and the ultrasound produced by the source transducer will have different frequencies. The receiver detects the difference between these two frequencies (the doppler shift) and drives a loudspeaker at this difference frequency. The doppler shift is typically one thousandth of the source frequency, which puts it in the audible range.

A continuous-wave instrument will detect flow that occurs anywhere within the intersection of the transmit and receive beams of the dual-transducer assembly. The doppler sample volume (the region from which doppler-shifted echoes return and are presented audibly or visually) is the overlapping region of the transmit and receive beams.

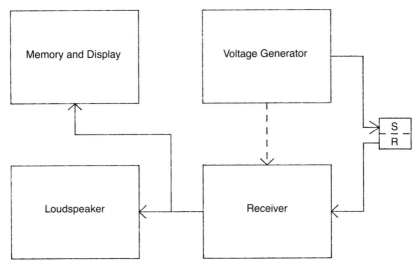

Figure 6.4. Block diagram of continuous-wave doppler instrument. The voltage generator produces a continuously alternating voltage that drives the source transducer (S). The receiving transducer (R) produces continuous voltage in response to reflections it continuously receives. The receiver detects any difference in frequency between the voltages produced by the continuous-wave generator and by the receiving transducer. The doppler shift produces a voltage that drives a loudspeaker in the audible range and a visual display. The frequency of the audible sound is equal to the doppler shift. It is proportional to the reflector speed and to the cosine of the angle between the sound propagation direction and the boundary motion (Section 6.2).

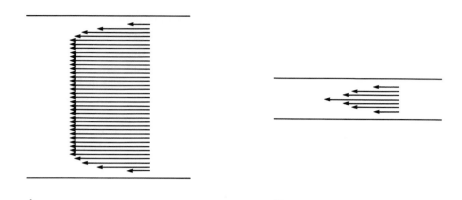

A   **B**

Figure 6.5. The flow profile is more uniform in a large-diameter vessel (a) than it is in a small one (b). (From Kremkau, F.W.: *In* Grant, E.G., and White, E.M.: Duplex Sonography. New York, Springer-Verlag, 1988. Reprinted with permission.)

Continuous-wave doppler systems can give motion artifacts if reflectors with different motions are included in the sound beams (e.g., two blood vessels being viewed simultaneously). Pulsed doppler systems help solve this problem by monitoring reflectors at selected distances or depths.

Because a distribution of flow velocities is encountered by the sound pulses as they traverse a vessel (Fig. 6.5), a distribution of many doppler-shifted frequencies returns to the transducer and the instrument (Fig. 6.6). As a presentation like Figure 6.6 is continuously changing with cardiac cycle, it can be displayed as a function of time with appropriate frequency spectrum processing (Figs. 6.7 and 6.8). These displays provide

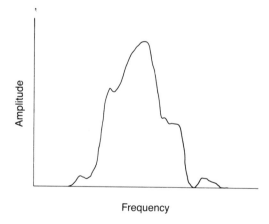

Figure 6.6. A frequency spectrum plot of the amplitude of each frequency component present in the returned pulses. Many frequencies are present because of the distribution of flow speeds encountered by the beam in the vessel.

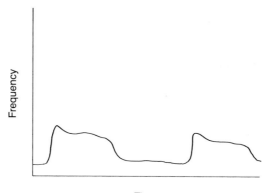

Time

Figure 6.7. A display of spectrum as a function of time (cardiac cycle). Frequency is now on the vertical axis. The amplitude of each frequency component at each instant of time is represented by gray level or color.

quantitative data for evaluating doppler-shifted echoes otherwise presented audibly. The fourier transform is the mathematical technique the instrument uses to derive the doppler spectrum from the returning echoes of various frequencies. These displays can show spectral broadening, which is the widening of the doppler shift spectrum, i.e., the increase of the range of doppler shift frequencies present, due to a broader range of flow speeds encountered by the sound beam. This occurs for normal flow in smaller vessels and for turbulent flow in any vessel.

It is important to realize that to correctly convert a spectral display from doppler shift versus time to flow speed versus time, the doppler angle must be accurately incorporated into the calculation process.

To eliminate the high-intensity low-frequency doppler shift echoes resulting from vessel wall motion during pulsatile flow, a high-pass filter (that rejects frequencies below an adjustable value) is used. Sometimes called a wall-thump filter, it rejects these strong echoes that would overwhelm the weaker echoes from the blood.

Exercises

6.3.1 All doppler instruments distinguish between positive and negative doppler shifts. True or false?

6.3.2 Instruments that distinguish between positive and negative doppler shifts yield motion _____ information and are called _____.

6.3.3 Continuous-wave doppler instruments use single-element transducers similar to those used in imaging. True or false?

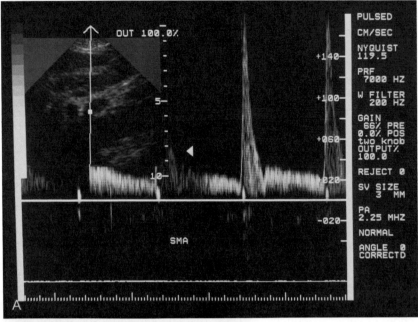

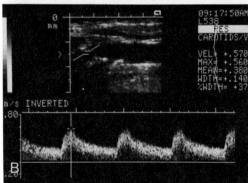

Figure 6.8. Clinical examples of a display of doppler spectrum as a function of time. (a) Superior mesenteric artery. (Courtesy of Advanced Technology Laboratories.) (b) Carotid artery. (Courtesy of Acuson.)

6.3.4 The components of a continuous-wave doppler system include
_____ _____, _____ _____,
_____ _____, _____, and _____.

6.3.5 Quantitative information about the frequencies contained in returning doppler-shifted echoes can be displayed on an _____ versus _____ plot that is continuously changing with time.

6.3.6 To display the pattern of time change of a doppler frequency spectrum, a display of _____ versus _____ can be used.

6.3.7 In Exercise 6.3.6, the amplitude of each frequency component is represented by _____ level or _____.

6.3.8 The received frequency spectrum exists (rather than a single frequency) because of the distribution of _____ _____ encountered by the pulse.

6.3.9 Because velocity is speed *and* direction, variations in either of these in the flow region monitored by the doppler instrument may contribute to the received frequency spectrum. True or false?

6.4
Pulsed-Wave Instruments

A diagram of the components of a pulsed doppler (pulsed wave) instrument is given in Figure 6.9. The voltage generator is similar to that in

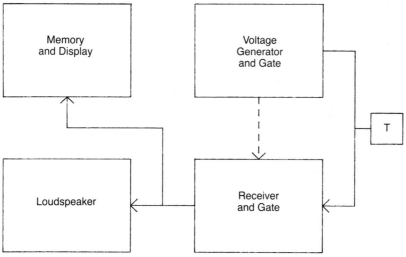

Figure 6.9. Block diagram of pulsed doppler instrument. The voltage generator produces a continuously alternating voltage. The generator gate converts this continuous voltage to voltage pulses that drive the transducer (T). This is normally a single-element transducer. Received pulses are delivered to the receiver, where their frequency is compared with the generator frequency. The difference (doppler shift) is sent to the loudspeaker and display. The receiver also contains a gate that selects reflections from a given depth according to arrival time and thus gives motion information as a function of depth. (From Kremkau, F.W.: *In* Grant, E.G., and White, E.M.: Duplex Sonography. New York, Springer-Verlag, 1988. Reprinted with permission.)

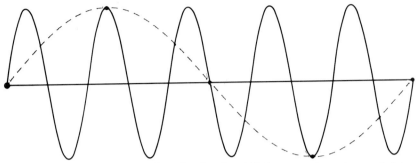

Figure 6.10. Aliasing occurs when the doppler shift frequency is undersampled in a pulsed system. Here only one sample (•) occurs each cycle, resulting in derived frequency (dashed line) much lower than the true doppler shift (solid line). (From Kremkau, F.W.: *In* Grant, E.G., and White, E.M.: Duplex Sonography. New York, Springer-Verlag, 1988. Reprinted with permission.)

Figure 6.4. The generator gate allows pulses of a few cycles of voltage to pass on to the transducer where ultrasound pulses are produced. As discussed in Chapter 2, imaging pulses are two or three cycles long. Pulses used in pulsed doppler instruments, however, have minimum pulse lengths of about five cycles. This is necessary to properly determine doppler shift of returning echoes. Pulses may be as long as 25 or 30 cycles. The transducer assembly normally contains only one transducer element, which functions as both the source and receiving transducer. Voltage pulses resulting from received reflections are processed in the receiver. The frequency of the pulses is compared with the voltage generator frequency, and the doppler shift is derived. It is sent to the loudspeaker for an audible output. Based on the arrival time of reflections (range equation; Section 2.5), those coming from reflectors at a

Table 6.4
Aliasing and Range-Ambiguity Artifact Values

Pulse Repetition Frequency (kHz)	Doppler Shift Above Which Aliasing Occurs (kHz)	Range Beyond Which Ambiguity Occurs (cm)
2.5	1.2	30
5.0	2.5	15
7.5	3.7	10
10.0	5.0	7
12.5	6.2	6
15.0	7.5	5
17.5	8.7	4
20.0	10.0	3
25.0	12.5	3
30.0	15.0	2

Table 6.5
Echo Arrival Time (t) for Various Reflector Depths (d)

d (cm)	t (μs)
0.5	6.5
1.0	13.0
2.0	26.0
4.0	52.0
8.0	104.0
15.0	195.0
20.0	260.0

(From Kremkau, F.W.: Technical considerations, equipment, and physics of duplex sonography. *In* Grant, E.G., and White, E.M.: Duplex Sonography. New York, Springer-Verlag, 1988. Reprinted with permission.)

given depth may be selected by the receiver gate; thus, motion information may be obtained as a function of depth. Receiver gate length and location (depth into tissue) are controllable by the operator. There is an upper limit to doppler shift that can be detected by pulsed instruments, which is one half the pulse repetition frequency (in the range of 5 to 30 kHz). When this limit (sometimes called the nyquist limit) is exceeded, aliasing occurs (Fig. 6.10). Improper doppler shift information (improper direction and improper value) results. An analogous optical form of aliasing occurs in motion pictures when wagon wheels appear to rotate at various speeds in reverse direction. Higher pulse repetition frequencies permit higher doppler shifts to be detected but also increase the chance of range ambiguity artifact (see Section 5.5 and Table 6.4). Continuous-wave doppler instruments do not have this limitation (but neither do they provide any depth information).

A single receiver gate selects one listening depth from which returning doppler-shifted echoes are accepted (Table 6.5). The gate has some

Table 6.6
Spatial Gate Length (L) for Various Temporal Gate Lengths (T)*

T (μs)	L (mm)
1.3	1
2.6	2
6.5	5
13.0	10

*Time from gate turn-on to turn-off. This table assumes zero pulse length. From Kremkau, F.W.: Technical considerations, equipment, and physics of duplex sonography. *In* Grant E.G., and White, E.M.: Duplex Sonography. New York, Springer-Verlag, 1988. Reprinted with permission.

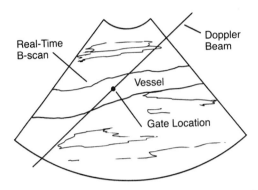

Figure 6.11. Image from a combined real-time and pulsed-doppler instrument. The doppler receiver gate can be located visually inside a vessel. Figure 6.8 shows such images from the displays of pulsed-wave instruments (sector and linear).

length (depth range) over which it permits reception (Table 6.6). For example (using the range equation: 13 μs round-trip travel time per centimeter of depth—Section 2.5), a gate that passes echoes arriving from 13 to 15 μs after pulse generation is effectively listening at a depth range of 10.0 to 11.6 mm. In this case the gate is located at a depth of 10.8 mm with a length (depth range) of ± 0.8 mm. A single gate allows only one depth and length selection (from which all doppler-shifted echoes will be accepted in combination) at any time. To simultaneously receive and separate doppler information from several depths (e.g., to obtain a flow profile across a vessel), multiple gates must be used. These separate the doppler information from several depths into separate channels for processing and display. The doppler sample volume (the region from which doppler-shifted echoes return and are presented audibly or visually) is determined by the beam width, the receiver gate length, and the pulse length.

Combinations of instruments discussed in Chapters 4 and 6 are available commercially. Pulsed and continuous-wave doppler systems are available in the same instrument. Real-time cross-sectional

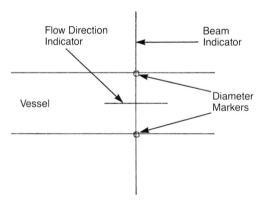

Figure 6.12. A duplex-doppler instrument display usually has operator-controllable indicators for flow direction and vessel diameter. (From Kremkau, F.W.: *In* Grant, E.G., and White, E.M.: Duplex Sonography. New York, Springer-Verlag, 1988. Reprinted with permission.)

ultrasound imaging instruments are available with continuous-wave and/or pulsed doppler. These provide the capability of imaging anatomic structure as well as analyzing motion and flow at a known point in the anatomic field (Figs. 6.8 and 6.11). The availability of continuous-wave and pulsed doppler in the same system is useful because difficulty is encountered in a pulsed system if the flow rates become so high that the doppler shift exceeds half the pulse repetition frequency (aliasing). At that point, the ability to shift to the continuous-wave system (even though it means giving up depth information) is advantageous.

Volume flow (mL/s) can be calculated from mean speed multiplied by vessel cross-sectional area. To do this correctly, the various doppler shifts representing the cells moving at various speeds must be averaged properly, the angle properly accounted for to convert mean doppler shift to mean speed, and area correctly determined from a vessel diameter measurement aided by the operator (Fig. 6.12) and assuming circular cross-section. Obviously several things could go wrong in this process, yielding faulty results.

Exercises

6.4.1 The components of a pulsed doppler instrument are the same as those for a continuous-wave instrument except for the addition of two _____ and the combining of two _____ into one.

6.4.2 The purpose of the generator gate is to convert a _____ voltage to a _____voltage.

6.4.3 The purpose of the receiver gate is to allow selection of doppler-shifted echoes from specific _____ according to _____ _____.

6.4.4 Pulsed doppler instruments require a two-element transducer assembly. True or false?

6.4.5 Multiple gates provide motion or flow _____ information.

6.4.6 The pulsed-doppler imaging instrument gives a cross-sectional display of motion and flow as a function of depth in tissue. True or false?

6.4.7 There is no problem with aliasing as long as the doppler shifts are _____ half the pulse repetition frequency.
   a. less than
   b. equal to
   c. greater than
   d. all of the above
   e. none of the above

6.4.8 To simultaneously receive and display doppler information from several depths, several _____ must be used in the receiver.

6.5
Color-Flow Instruments

The continuous-wave and pulsed-wave instruments described in the previous two sections are limited to a presentation of real-time doppler-shift information from a relatively localized region within tissue. As discussed previously, this is normally presented as a plot of doppler shift versus time. It is desirable to display doppler flow information in a manner similar to real-time sonography of anatomic structures. This is accomplished using a pulse-echo technique similar to that for gray-scale imaging. That is, pulses are sent through all regions of the anatomic field from which flow information is desired. But rather than displaying returning echoes with gray-scale brightnesses corresponding to their intensities, as in anatomic imaging, echoes are displayed with colors corresponding to the direction of flow that their positive or negative doppler shifts represent (toward or away from the transducer). The brightness of the color represents the intensity of the echoes, and sometimes other colors are added to indicate the extent of spectral broadening. Color choices for these applications are not standardized, and there is some debate regarding which are best.

The rapid rate of echo return and presentation on the display does not permit determination of the doppler spectrum using the fourier transform technique. Instead, an autocorrelation technique is used. Each echo is correlated with the corresponding one from the previous pulse, thus determining the motion that has occurred during each pulse period. A real-time value for mean flow speed is yielded. As this is positive or negative with respect to flow direction, it is possible to present real-time color-coded flow direction information two-dimensionally on the display. This is normally superimposed on the two-dimensional gray-scale anatomic scan. Examples are given in Figures 6.13 to 6.15. The aliasing artifact appears in these displays as a region of different color (opposite flow) where the doppler shift exceeds half the pulse repetition frequency (Fig. 6.16).

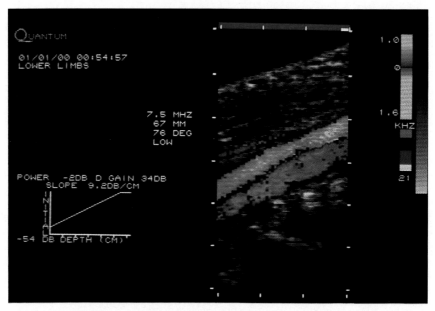

Figure 6.13. Clinical example of color-flow doppler showing opposite flow directions in the two vessels. (Courtesy of Quantum Medical Systems.)

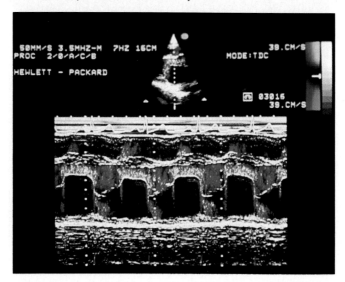

Figure 6.14. Clinical example of color-flow doppler combined with M mode in the heart. (Courtesy of Hewlett Packard.)

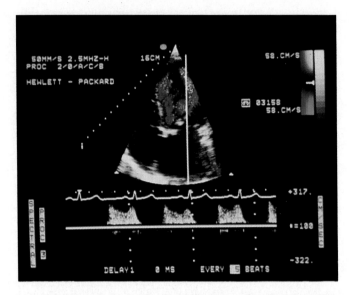

Figure 6.15. Clinical example of color-flow doppler combined with continuous-wave doppler spectrum in the heart. (Courtesy of Hewlett Packard.)

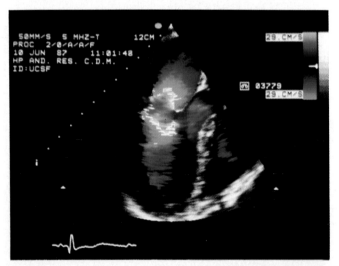

Figure 6.16. Transesophageal cardiac color-flow image of the long axis in diastole. The blue colors between the left atrium and left ventricle represent blood traveling away from the transducer, but because of very high velocities, aliasing has occurred and the yellow and orange colors have replaced the blue colors. (Courtesy of Hewlett Packard.)

Exercises

6.5.1 Color-flow instruments present two-dimensional color-coded images representing _____ that are superimposed on gray-scale images representing _____.

6.5.2 Which of the following on a color-flow display is (are) presented in real-time?
   a. gray-scale anatomy
   b. flow direction
   c. doppler spectrum
   d. a and b
   e. all of the above

6.5.3 If red represents flow toward the transducer and blue represents flow away, what color would be seen for normal flow toward the transducer? What color would be seen for aliasing flow toward the transducer? What colors for normal flow away and for aliasing flow away?

6.5.4 Color-flow instruments use an _____ technique to yield _____ flow speed in real-time.

6.5.5 The fourier-transform technique is not used in color-flow instruments because it is not _____ enough.
   a. slow
   b. fast
   c. bright
   d. cheap
   e. none of the above

6.6
Review

The doppler effect is a change in frequency resulting from reflector or scatterer motion toward or away from the source. Doppler instruments make use of this frequency shift to yield information regarding motion and flow. Continuous-wave systems provide motion and flow information without depth information or selection capability. Pulsed doppler systems provide depth information and the ability to select depth at which doppler information is generated. Spectral analysis provides information on the distribution of received frequencies resulting from the distribution of scatterer velocities encountered. In addition to audible output, imaging of vessel flow spectra is possible in doppler systems. Combined systems utilizing dynamic B-scan imaging and continuous-wave and pulsed doppler are available commercially. Color-flow systems provide displays of two-dimensional, real-time flow superimposed on gray-scale anatomic scans.

Definitions of terms used in this chapter are listed below:

Aliasing. Improper doppler shift information from a pulsed-doppler instrument when true doppler shift exceeds half the pulse repetition frequency.

Autocorrelation. A rapid technique for obtaining mean doppler shift frequency. This technique is used in color-flow instruments.

Bidirectional. Indicating doppler instruments capable of distinguishing between positive and negative doppler shifts (forward and reverse flow).

Color-flow. The presentation of two-dimensional, real-time doppler shift information superimposed on a real-time, gray-scale anatomic cross-sectional image. Flow directions toward and away from the transducer, i.e., positive and negative doppler shifts, are presented as different colors on the display.

Cosine. The cosine of angle A in Figure C.1 (Appendix C) is the length of side b divided by the length of side c.

Doppler angle. The angle between the sound beam and flow direction.

Doppler effect. Frequency change of reflected sound wave as a result of reflector motion relative to transducer.

Doppler shift. Reflected frequency minus incident frequency.

Fourier transform. A mathematical technique for obtaining a doppler frequency spectrum.

Frequency spectrum. The range of frequencies present. In a doppler instrument, the range of doppler shift frequencies present in the returning echoes.

Generator gate. The electronic portion of a pulsed doppler system that converts the continuous voltage of the voltage generator to a pulsed voltage.

Receiver gate. A device that allows only echoes from a selected depth (arrival time) to pass.

Spectral broadening. The widening of the doppler shift spectrum, i.e. the increase of the range of doppler shift frequencies present, due to a broader range of flow speeds encountered by the sound beam. This occurs for normal flow in smaller vessels and for turbulent flow in any vessel.

Exercises

6.6.1 Doppler systems convert _____ _____ information to audible sound or visual display.

6.6.2 A pulser similar to that used in imaging systems is used in doppler systems. True or false?

6.6.3 Doppler system transducers may have _____ or _____ elements.

6.6.4 The receiver in a doppler system compares the _____ of the voltage generator and the voltage from the receiving transducer.

6.6.5 The doppler shift usually is not in the audible frequency range and must be converted by the receiver to a frequency that can be heard. True or false?

6.6.6 Doppler shift is determined by reflector _____ and by the cosine of an angle.

6.6.7 A component that pulsed doppler systems have but continuous-wave doppler systems do not have is the _____.

6.6.8 A doppler system may have as an output a visual _____.

6.6.9 In a pulsed doppler system, the pulse repetition frequency is determined by the generator _____, and the source ultrasound frequency is determined by the _____.

6.6.10 Pulsed doppler systems can give motion information as a function of _____.

6.6.11 A typical SPTA output intensity for a doppler instrument is 10 mW/cm^2. True or false?

6.6.12 The sound received by the transducer in a doppler instrument is in the audible frequency range. True or false?

6.6.13 Frequencies used in doppler ultrasound are in approximately the same range as those for pulse echo imaging. True or false?

6.6.14 If the incident frequency is 4 MHz, the reflector speed is 100 cm/s, and the angle between beam and motion directions is 60 degrees, the doppler shift is _____ kHz.

6.6.15. There is no problem in Exercise 6.6.14 with aliasing with a pulse frequency of 10 kHz. True or false?

6.6.16. If there were a problem in Exercise 6.6.15, _____ doppler ultrasound could be used to avoid it.

6.6.17. Color-flow instruments use
  a. continuous-wave doppler
  b. pulsed doppler
  c. compressed doppler
  d. all of the above
  e. none of the above

Chapter 7

Performance and Safety

7.1
Introduction

This chapter deals with two topics. First, devices and methods are used to determine if diagnostic ultrasound imaging instruments are operating correctly and consistently. These devices and methods are considered in three groups: (1) those that test the operation of the instrument as a whole (imaging performance); (2) those that measure the beams produced by transducers; and (3) those that measure the acoustic output of the instrument. Group 1 takes into account the operations of all the components shown in Figure 4.2. Group 2 considers only the transducer. Group 3 considers only the pulser and the transducer acting as a source. In group 2 tests, the transducer is driven and evaluated by a separate test generator or by the diagnostic instrument. Imaging performance is important for evaluating the instrument as a diagnostic tool. Beam profiles are important when evaluating and choosing transducers. The acoustic output of an instrument is important when considering bioeffects and safety, which is the second topic of this chapter.

Bioeffects are useful in therapeutic applications of ultrasound, a subject not considered here. Of concern is what the bioeffects of ultrasound tell us about the safety or hazard of diagnostic ultrasound. What would be desirable would be to ask the question, "Is it safe?" and to give the answer, "Yes." If this were possible, several pages on the subject would not be needed. This ideal situation is not necessary for the procedure to be useful, however. Such a strong criterion is not applied to other areas of life. It cannot be said that riding in a car is safe; yet we choose to go off in one daily. What is desirable is knowledge of the probability of damage or injury and under what conditions this probability is maximized (in order to avoid those conditions) and minimized (in order to seek those conditions).

In this chapter we consider the following questions: How do we determine whether or not an imaging or doppler instrument is working properly or not? What devices are available for testing various performance characteristics of instruments? What is the difference between a test object and a phantom? Are there any known risks in the use of imaging or doppler ultrasound? How can an operator of an ultrasound instrument minimize exposure of the patient to ultrasound? The following terms are discussed in this chapter:

beam profiler

cavitation

dead zone

hydrophone

phantom

test object

7.2
Imaging Performance

Imaging performance is determined by measuring the following parameters:

1. system sensitivity and dynamic range
2. contrast resolution (Section 4.4)
3. detail resolution (Section 3.5)
4. dead zone

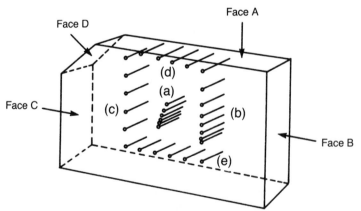

Figure 7.1. The AIUM 100-mm test object. Rod groups are used for measuring (a) axial resolution, (b) or (c) lateral resolution, (c) range accuracy and receiver compensation, (d) dead zone, and (a) through (e) registration accuracy. Any rod imaged may be used for sensitivity or dynamic range measurements.

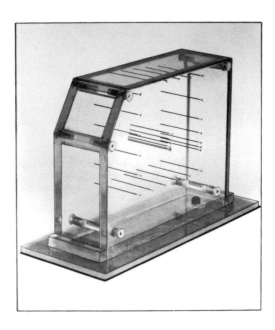

Figure 7.2. A commercial version of the AIUM test object. (Courtesy of Nuclear Associates).

5. range (depth or distance) accuracy (Sections 2.5 and 4.5)
6. compensation (swept gain) operation (Section 4.3)

These may all be measured using the 100-mm test object of the American Institute of Ultrasound in Medicine (AIUM) (Fig. 7.1). This test object is composed of a series of 0.75-mm diameter stainless-steel rods arranged in a pattern between two transparent plastic sides. The other sides are made of thin acrylic plastic sheets on which the transducer may be placed using a coupling medium. The tank is filled with a mixture of alcohol, algae inhibitor, and water that has a propagation speed of 1.54 mm/µs at room temperature. The speed varies by less than 1 per cent when the temperature is changed by 5°C. Therefore, results with this test object are relatively insensitive to normal fluctuations in room temperature. Construction details and procedures for its use have been published.[22-23] These test objects are available commercially (Fig. 7.2).

To obtain consistent measurements of axial and lateral resolution and dead zone, even with a given transducer and diagnostic instrument, it is necessary to perform the test at consistent control settings. Usually it is best to measure relative system sensitivity first and then increase the sensitivity settings a fixed amount for performing the other tests.

Relative system sensitivity is a measure of how weak a reflection an instrument can display. It is obtained by finding the gain or attenuation setting (with no compensation) at which a particular rod in the test object produces a barely discernible display. Any imaged rod may be chosen for

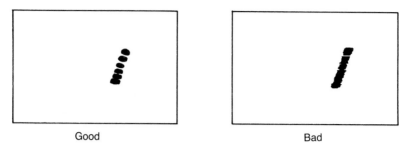

Figure 7.3.   Axial resolution. Rod group (a) in Figure 7.1 is used. Separations from 1 to 5 mm may be viewed. On the left, axial resolution is 1 or 2 mm. On the right, it is 5 mm. Figure 3.23 gives examples of scans with this rod group.

this measurement. Usually the top rod in group (a) or the bottom rod in group (c) is used for system sensitivity measurements (Fig. 7.1). For the remaining measurements, 10 dB are added to the system sensitivity settings required to barely display the chosen rod.

Axial resolution is measured with rod group (a). The transducer is placed on face A above the rod group. Not all the rods will be seen separately on the display. The spacing of the two closest rods in the group that are seen separately on the display is equal to the axial resolution (Fig. 3.23 and 7.3). Axial resolution measured with the test object usually does not reflect the best possible resolution of the diagnostic system. The measurement, however, is a consistency check for use with a given transducer and instrument.

Lateral resolution is measured with rod group (b). The transducer is scanned along face B. Not all the rods will be seen separately on the display. The spacing of the two closest rods in the group that are seen separately on the display is equal to the lateral resolution (Fig. 7.4[a]). Lateral resolution at a range from 1 to 11 cm can be determined by measuring the width of the line representing each rod in group (c) after the transducer is scanned across face A of the test object ([Fig. 7.4[b]).

The dead zone is the distance closest to the transducer in which imaging cannot be performed. It is measured with rod group (d). The transducer is scanned across face A. The distance from the transducer to the first rod imaged is equal to the dead zone.

Range accuracy is measured with rod group (c). The rods should appear on the display at 1, 3, 5, 7, 9, and 11 cm from the transducer (Fig. 7.5). Relative distances between the rods should be accurate to at least 2 mm or less. The space between the rods at 1 and 11 cm should be recorded with calipers and then measured with marker dots placed parallel to rod group (e). If this indicates that the distance between the

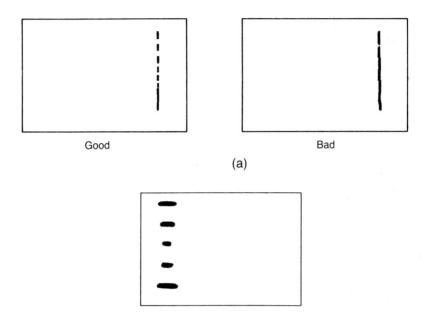

Good   Bad

(a)

(b)

Figure 7.4. Lateral resolution. (a) Using rod group (b) in Figure 7.1, separations from 3 to 25 mm may be viewed. On the left, lateral resolution is about 5 mm. On the right it is about 25 mm. (b) Using rod group (c) in Figure 7.1, the widths of rod images at various depths give lateral resolutions at these depths. A segmented picture of the beam is also presented with this view.

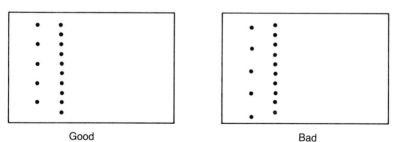

Good   Bad

Figure 7.5. Range accuracy is tested using rod group (c) in Figure 7.1. The rods should appear with 2-cm separations as on the left. One-centimeter marker dots are displayed here as well.

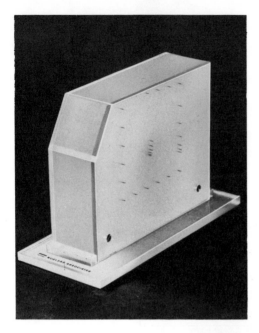

Figure 7.6. AIUM test object filled with tissue-equivalent material. (Courtesy of Nuclear Associates.)

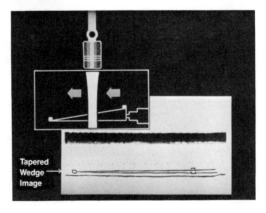

Figure 7.7. A commercial version of the SUAR test object. (Courtesy of Nuclear Associates.)

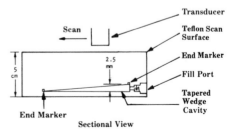

Sector Scan Phantom

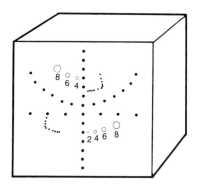

Model 515

Figure 7.8. Commercial tissue-equivalent phantom containing wires and echo-free (cystic) areas. (Courtesy of ATS Laboratories.)

rods at 1 and 11 cm differs from the true 10 cm by more than 2 mm, then the horizontal and vertical display scales are not identical.

Compensation operation is measured using rod group (c). The transducer is placed on face A above this rod group. With no compensation, the attenuator or gain settings required to display each rod at a given pulse height (A mode) or gray level (B or M mode) are recorded. This is then done again with compensation on. The difference between the settings for each rod as a function of distance is the compensation characteristic.

The gray-scale dynamic range is the difference between gain or attenuator settings (dB) that produce (1) barely discernible and (2) maximum deflection (A mode) or brightness (B or M mode) displays for the same reflection. Any rod imaged may be chosen for this measurement.

Several other objects are available commercially for testing imaging performance. These fall into two categories: test objects (e.g., the AIUM test object discussed earlier) and tissue-equivalent (TE) phantoms. Tissue-equivalent phantoms have some characteristics representative of tissues (e.g., scattering or attenuation properties), whereas test objects do not. Some objects are combinations of the two (e.g., an AIUM test object filled with tissue-equivalent medium rather than a water-alcohol mixture) (Fig. 7.6). The sensitivity, uniformity, and axial resolution (SUAR) test object uses a wedge cavity in a block to allow axial resolution measurement over a continuous range of separations (Fig. 7.7). Tissue-equivalent phantoms containing echo-free (cystic) regions (Fig. 7.8), scattering layers for scattered beam profile visualization (Figs. 3.24[b], 3.25[b] and 7.9), arrays of echo-free cylinders of various radii at various

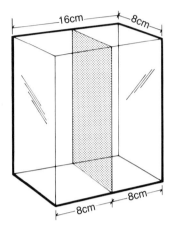

Model 508

Figure 7.9.   Commercial version of beam-profile test object. (Courtesy of ATS Laboratories.) Scans with such a test object are shown in Figures 3.24(b) and 3.25(b).

depths (Figs. 3.24[a], 3.25[a] and 7.10), cones and cylinders containing material of various scattering strengths (Fig. 7.11), or blocks of various scattering materials (gray-scale levels) are available (Fig. 7.12).

The particle image resolution test object (PIRTO) is filled with polystyrene spheres randomly distributed in a low-attenuation, low-scatter gel (Fig. 7.13).

In addition to test objects and phantoms designed for imaging performance evaluation, devices are also available for doppler system evaluation (Fig. 7.14).

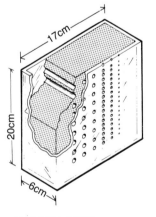

Model 504 & 534

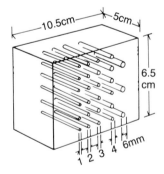

Model 506 & 536

Figure 7.10.   Commercial versions of resolution-penetration phantoms. (Courtesy of ATS Laboratories.)

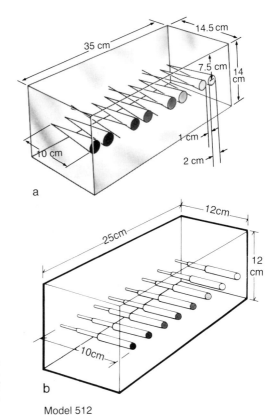

a

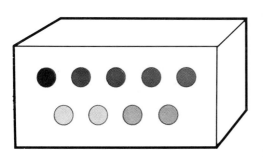

b

Figure 7.11. Commercial versions of contrast/detail resolution phantoms. (a), Courtesy of Nuclear Associates; and (b), courtesy of ATS Laboratories.)

Model 512

Model 531

Figure 7.12. Commercial version of gray-scale test phantom. (Courtesy of ATS Laboratories.)

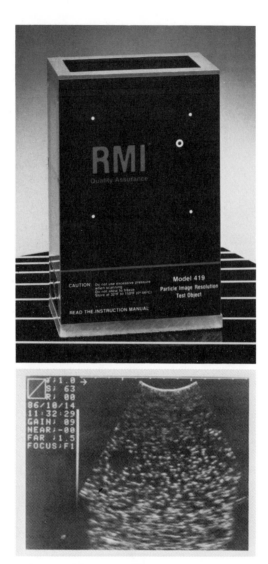

**PARTICLE IMAGE RESOLUTION TEST OBJECT
MODEL 419**

Figure 7.13.   Commercial version of a PIRTO phantom. (Courtesy of RMI.)

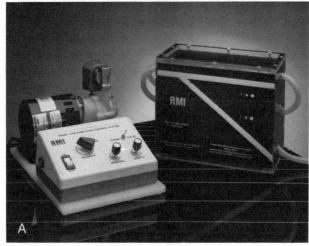

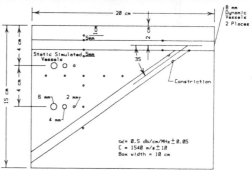

Figure 7.14. Commercial doppler phantom and flow system.
(Courtesy of RMI.) B

**Schematic of Model 409A
Doppler Phantom**

The AIUM test object described in this section measures one beam parameter, the beam diameter, which is equal to lateral resolution. However, it does this only at one distance from the transducer: the distance from face B to rod group (b) in Figure 7.1. The use of rod group (c) in Figure 7.1 does not suffer from this same restriction. However, there is some distortion of the lateral resolution measurements in rod group (c) because of shadowing of lower rods by rods in the focal region. The test object is used to make this measurement using the ultrasound imaging instrument as a whole (the rod reflections are imaged on the instrument display). Scattering-layer test objects (Figs. 3.24[b], 3.25[b], and 7.9) provide qualitative beam presentations. A beam profiler is a device designed to give three-dimensional (quantitative) reflection amplitude information. It uses rods at various distances from the

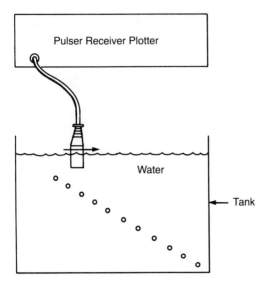

Figure 7.15. A beam profiler consists of a pulser, receiver, plotter, transducer, and tank with rods at various distances from the transducer. The transducer is scanned over the rods.

transducer (Fig. 7.15). The transducer is pulsed as it is scanned across the tank. Reflections are received from each rod, and voltage amplitude is measured. As the sound beam passes over a rod, the reflected amplitude increases, goes through a maximum, and then decreases. Then the next rod (at a greater distance) is encountered, with a similar reflection behavior. This continues until all rods have been encountered. A beam profile can be plotted from this procedure (Fig. 7.16). A beam profile does

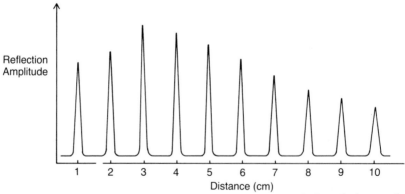

Figure 7.16. Beam profile plotted by the system in Figure 7.15. Each peak shows reflection amplitude as scanned across the rod that is at the distance indicated from the transducer. The amplitude is maximum at the near-zone length of an unfocused transducer or at the focal region of a focused transducer (Section 4.3).

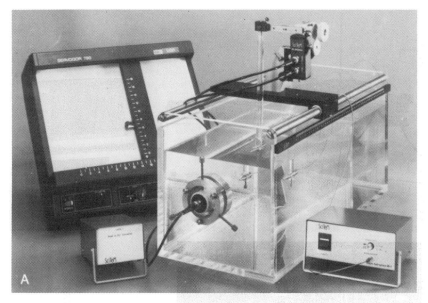

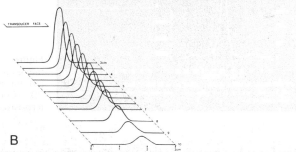

Figure 7.17. Hydrophone system (A) for measuring beam profile (B) (Courtesy of Medisonics.)

not actually give a profile of a beam, i.e., it does not plot acoustic amplitude or intensity across the beam at several distances from the transducer as it appears to do. It actually plots reflection amplitude received at the transducer, and it could be called a reflection profiler. For imaging instruments, however, this profile is a useful thing. Such profiles are often supplied with transducers to show beam characteristics obtained by this method. Hydrophones (Section 7.3) can also be beam profilers in that they can measure pressure and intensity distributions across beams (Figs. 7.17 and 7.18).

Pulses produced by ultrasound transducers contain a range of frequencies called the bandwidth (Section 3.2). Transducer specifications

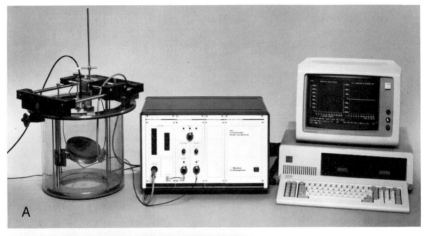

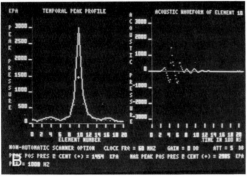

Figure 7.18. Linear array membrane hydrophone system (A) for measuring beam profile (B). (Courtesy of Nuclear Enterprises.)

often include a picture of the frequency spectrum of the pulses produced. This is a plot of amplitude (of each frequency component) versus frequency (Fig. 3.6). It is obtained by receiving the pulse with a hydrophone or with the same transducer that produced it (after reflection from a sphere, rod, or plate). The electric pulse from the hydrophone or transducer is sent to a spectrum analyzer, which breaks it down into its component frequencies and displays them.

Exercises

7.2.1 The 100-mm test object contains several stainless steel _____ immersed in a mixture of algae inhibitor, _____, and _____ that has a propagation speed of 1.54 mm/µs.

7.2.2 Match the parameters measured with the rod groups used (Fig. 7.1) (answers may be used more than once):

a. axial resolution: _____   1. rod group (a)
b. lateral resolution: _____   2. rod group (b)
c. range accuracy: _____   3. rod group (c)
d. registration accuracy: 4. rod group (d)
_____   5. rod group (e)
e. dead zone: _____   6. all rods
f. compensation: _____   7. any rod
g. sensitivity: _____
h. dynamic range: _____

7.2.3 Match the parameters measured with the types of observation modes (answers may be used more than once):

a. axial resolution: _____   1. gain or attenuator settings
b. lateral resolution: _____   2. first rod imaged
c. range accuracy: _____   3. rod distances from transducer
d. dead zone: _____   in the display
e. compensation: _____   4. minimum spacing of separately
f. sensitivity: _____   displayed rods
g. dynamic range: _____

7.2.4 Test objects are available commercially. True or false?

7.2.5 Results using a test object are relatively insensitive to temperature. True or false?

7.2.6 The speed of sound in the recommended alcohol and water mixture of the AIUM test object varies by less than _____ per cent when the temperature is changed by 5°C.

7.2.7 A limitation to the use of rod group (b) for lateral resolution measurement is that it yields an observation at only one _____ from the transducer.

7.2.8 To solve the difficulty in Exercise 7.2.7, rod group (c) may be used to yield beam width information at several _____.

7.2.9 Tissue-equivalent phantoms attempt to represent some acoustic property of _____.

7.2.10 The AIUM test object is an example of a TE phantom. True or false?

7.2.11 Which of these devices measure(s) parameters related to beam profiling?

a. 100-mm test object
b. SUAR test object
c. hydrophone
d. both a and c
e. both b and c

7.2.12 Reflection profilers plot acoustic amplitude or intensity across the beam at several distances from the transducer. True or false?

7.2.13 The following are often supplied with beam profiles to show their characteristics:
   a. pulsers
   b. transducers
   c. receivers
   d. displays
   e. both a and c

7.2.14 A spectrum analyzer is used to determine _____.
   a. color spectrum
   b. impedance spectrum
   c. lateral resolution
   d. frequency spectrum
   e. all of the above

7.3
Acoustic Output

Several devices can measure the acoustic output of ultrasound imaging instruments. Only one, the hydrophone, will be discussed here. The hydrophone is a small (1 mm in diameter or less) transducer element mounted on the end of a narrow tube or hollow needle (Fig. 7.19). Its size causes it to receive sound reasonably well from all directions without altering the sound by its presence. In response to the varying pressure of the sound, it produces a varying voltage that can be displayed on an

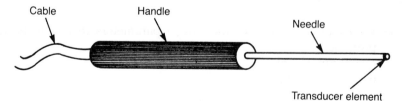

Figure 7.19.   A hydrophone consists of a small transducer element mounted on the end of a needle.

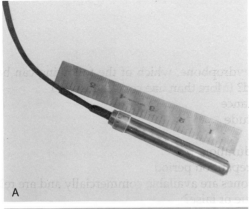

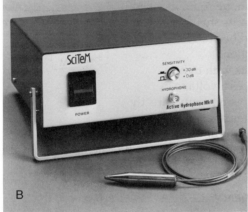

Figure 7.20. Commercial hydrophone. [(A), Courtesy of Nuclear Associates; (B), Courtesy of Medisonics.]

oscilloscope. A picture similar to that in Figure 2.15[a] is produced, from which period, pulse repetition period, and pulse duration can be determined. From these quantities, frequency, pulse repetition frequency, and duty factor can be calculated. If the hydrophone calibration is known (relationship between voltage produced and pressure applied), pressure amplitude may also be determined. If propagation speed is known, wavelength and spatial pulse length can be calculated (Sections 2.2 and 2.3). If impedance is known, intensity can be calculated. Hydrophones are available commercially (Fig. 7.20) and are relatively inexpensive and simple to use. Polyvinylidene fluoride (PVDF) is the thin film material commonly used in modern hydrophones.

Exercises

7.3.1 Using a hydrophone, which of the following can be measured or calculated? (More than one correct answer.)
   a. impedance
   b. amplitude
   c. period
   d. pulse duration
   e. pulse repetition period
7.3.2 Hydrophones are available commercially and are relatively simple to use. True or false?
7.3.3 A hydrophone contains a small _____ element.
7.3.4 Because of its small size, a hydrophone can measure spatial details of a sound beam. True or false?
7.3.5 A hydrophone
   a. interacts with light
   b. produces a voltage
   c. measures intensity directly
   d. measures total energy
   e. none of the above
7.3.6 Match the following (A can be calculated from B if C is known) (answers may be used more than once):
   A:
      a. frequency: _____, _____
      b. pulse repetition frequency:_____, _____
      c. duty factor: _____, _____
      d. wavelength: _____, _____
      e. spatial pulse length:_____, _____
      f. power: _____, _____
      g. intensity: _____, _____

   B:
   1. wavelength
   2. period
   3. pulse repetition period
   4. frequency
   5. energy
   6. power

   C:
   7. number of cycles in the pulse
   8. pulse duration
   9. propagation speed
   10. exposure time
   11. beam area
   12. nothing else

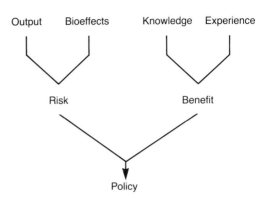

Figure 7.21. Ultrasound risk and benefit information. Risk information comes from experimental bioeffects, epidemiology, and instrument output data. Benefit information comes from knowledge and experience in ultrasound imaging use and efficacy. Together they lead to policy on the prudent use of ultrasound imaging in medicine.

7.4
Bioeffects

In any diagnostic test there may be some risk (some probability of damage or injury). For diagnostic ultrasound, the sonologist and sonographer need to know something about this risk. Risk can be weighed against benefit to determine the appropriateness of the diagnostic procedure (Fig. 7.21). Knowledge of how to minimize the risk is useful to everyone involved in diagnostic ultrasound.

There are several sources of bioeffects information (Fig. 7.22).

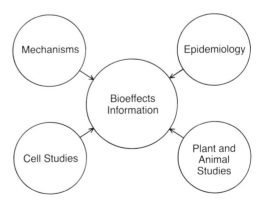

Figure 7.22. Bioeffects information sources.

However, a complete knowledge of the bioeffects of ultrasound is unavailable. What types of injury can diagnostic ultrasound produce in patients? Under what conditions? Sufficient epidemiologic data are not available.

What is known is something about bioeffects in experimental animals. Hundreds of reports on this subject can be found in the scientific literature. Several reviews of this subject have appeared.[24-30]

The American Institute of Ultrasound in Medicine (AIUM) has reviewed the reports of bioeffects in ultrasound and in 1987 issued the following statement:

In Vivo Mammalian Bioeffects
A review of bioeffects data supports the following statement as an update of the AIUM Statement on In Vivo Mammalian Bioeffects:

In the low megahertz frequency range there have been (as of this date) no independently confirmed significant biological effects in mammalian tissues exposed in vivo to unfocused ultrasound with intensities[a] below 100 mW/cm^2, or to focused ultrasound[b] with intensities below 1 W/cm^2. Furthermore, for exposure times[c] greater than 1 second and less than 500 seconds (for unfocused ultrasound) or 50 seconds (for focused ultrasound), such effects have not been demonstrated even at higher intensities, when the product of intensity and exposure time is less than 50 joules/cm^2.

---

[a] Free-field spatial peak, temporal average (SPTA) for continuous-wave exposures and for pulsed-mode exposures with pulses repeated at a frequency greater than 100 Hz.

[b] Quarter-power (–6dB) beam width smaller than four wavelengths or 4 mm, whichever is less at the exposure frequency.

[c] Total time includes off-time as well on-time for repeated pulse regimes.

The low-megahertz range referred to in this statement is 0.5 to 10 MHz. The intensity considered is the SPTA intensity discussed in Section 2.4. "Free field" means that there were no reflections from the walls of the measuring system. "Repeated-pulse regimes" (pulsed ultrasound) are discussed in Section 2.3. The product of intensity and time is

$$\text{intensity} \times \text{time} \quad = \quad \left[\frac{\text{power}}{\text{area}}\right] \times \left[\text{time}\right] \qquad \text{(Section 2.4)}$$

$$= \quad \left[\frac{\text{energy}}{\text{time}}\right] \times \left[\frac{\text{time}}{\text{area}}\right] \qquad \text{(Appendix D)}$$

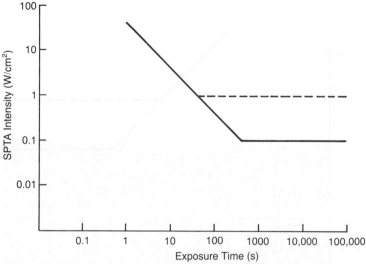

Figure 7.23. The intensity and time limits described by the AIUM statement on in vivo mammalian bioeffects. There are no independently confirmed significant bioeffects in mammalian tissues for intensity and time conditions below the line. Intensity is SPTA as measured in a free field in water. Time is total time of exposure to ultrasound (includes time between pulses in the case of pulsed ultrasound).

$$= \frac{energy}{area} \quad (J/cm^2) \qquad \text{(Table C.4, Appendix C)}$$

This is the energy passed through an area divided by the area.

This statement describes intensity and time limits below which "independently confirmed significant" bioeffects have not been reported. These limits are shown in Figure 7.23. They are probably not minimum or threshold levels. As more sensitive biologic endpoints are studied, it is reasonable to expect some lowering of these levels.

Reports used in determining the preceding statement considered the following bioeffects: hind-limb paralysis, fetal weight reduction, postpartum mortality, and liver mitotic index reduction, all in mice and rats; blood vessel damage in chick embryos; wound healing in rabbit ears; and postulated human fetal abnormalities based on absorption heating. The results were obtained with focused as well as unfocused beams, generated continuously or (to a lesser extent) as pulsed ultrasound.

A comparison of the instrument output data from Table 4.2 with the bioeffects statement levels is given in Figure 7.24. Pulsed doppler instrument outputs range as high as 2000 mW/cm^2. In making this comparison, the pulsed ultrasound of the instruments is compared with the continuous sound used in most bioeffects studies. This is done by using

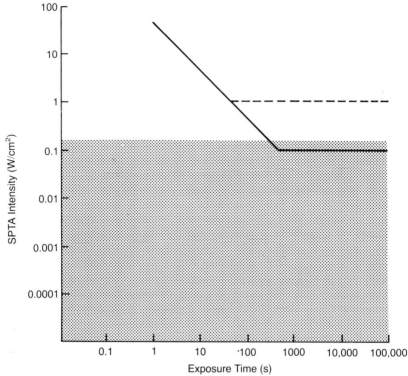

Figure 7.24.   A comparison of imaging instrument output data with the AIUM bioeffects statement level. The shaded area shows the range in which diagnostic instruments fall (Table 4.2). The SPTA intensity is used, assuming that temporal average is relevant. Time is total time of exposure to ultrasound (includes time between pulses in the case of pulsed ultrasound).

the SPTA intensity (see Section 2.4) of the pulsed ultrasound. If bioeffects depend on temporal average intensity, this is a valid comparison. Three mechanisms of action for ultrasound bioeffects are generally recognized:

1. heat
2. cavitation (production and behavior of bubbles in sound)
3. other

The third class is sometimes called mechanical. Little is known about it. For purposes here, it means nonthermal and noncavitational. Heating depends on temporal average intensity, cavitation does not. The intensity dependence of the category "other" is unknown.

   The AIUM has issued 1987 statements on these mechanisms as follows:

Thermal Mechanism

1. A thermal criterion is one reasonable approach to specifying potentially hazardous exposures for diagnostic ultrasound.

2. Based solely on a thermal criterion, a diagnostic exposure that produces a maximum temperature rise of 1°C above normal physiologic levels may be used in clinical examinations without reservation.

3. An in situ temperature rise to or above 41°C is considered hazardous in fetal exposures; the longer this temperature elevation is maintained, the greater the likelihood for damage to occur is.

4. Analytic models of ultrasonically induced heating have been applied successfully to in vivo mammalian situations. In those clinical situations in which local tissue temperatures are not measured, estimates of temperature elevations can be made by employing such analytic models.

5. Calculations of ultrasonically induced temperature elevation, based on a simplified tissue model and a simplified model of stationary beams, suggest the following: For examinations in soft fetal tissues with typical perfusion rates, employing center frequencies between 2 and 10 MHz and beam widths* less than 11 wavelengths, the computed temperature rise will not be significantly above 1°C if the in situ SATA intensity† does not exceed 200 mW/cm². If the beam width does not exceed eight wavelengths, the corresponding intensity is 300 mW/cm². However, if the same beam impinges on fetal bone the local temperature rise may be much higher.

---

*-6 dB beam width, according to AIUM/National Electrical Manufacturers Association definition.

†"SATA" = average over focal area.

Cavitation

1. Acoustic cavitation may occur with short pulses and has the potential for producing deleterious biologic effects.

2. Currently available information indicates that pulses with peak pressures greater than 10 MPa (3300 W/cm^2) can induce cavitation in mammals.*

3. With the limited data available, it is not possible to specify *threshold* pressure amplitudes at which acoustic cavitation will occur, in mammals, with diagnostically relevant pulse lengths and repetition rates.

---

*Evidence from observations with lithotripters.

The overlap in Figure 7.24 suggests that with the instruments that operate at the higher intensities, it may be possible to produce some bioeffects in small animals. The likelihood of this seems to be greatest for pulsed doppler, for which the SPTA outputs are the highest (as much as 2000 mW/cm). However, there is no evidence that bioeffects do occur in clinical use of any of these instruments.

Another consideration in these comparisons is whether or not sound exposures separated by several hours or days add up (repair or recovery does not occur between exposures). No data are available to permit any statement on this consideration.

Several reports have appeared in the literature that appear to violate the AIUM statement. They do not, however, either because they do not deal with mammalian tissues or because they have not been independently confirmed. Several of these reports have dealt with in vitro studies. The relevance of these to clinical imaging safety is weak, at best. This is described by the AIUM Statement on In Vitro Biological Effects (March 1988).[26]

Statement on In Vitro Biological Effects
It is difficult to evaluate reports of ultrasonically induced in vitro biological effects with respect to their clinical significance. The predominant physical and biological interactions and mechanisms involved in an in vitro effect may not pertain to the in vivo situation. Nevertheless, an in vitro effect must be regarded as a real biological effect.

Results from in vitro experiments suggest new endpoints and serve as a basis for design of in vivo experiments. In vitro studies provide the capability to control experimental variables and thus offer a means to explore and evaluate specific mechanisms. Although they may have limited applicability to in vivo biological effects, such studies can disclose fundamental intercellular or intracellular interactions. While it is valid for authors to place their results in context and to suggest further relevant investigations, reports of in vitro studies which claim direct clinical significance should be viewed with caution.

The AIUM Biological Effects Committee continually reviews published articles relevant to ultrasound safety and publishes short critiques.

Exercises

7.4.1 Heating depends most directly on
  a. SATA intensity
  b. SATP intensity
  c. SPTP intensity
7.4.2 When SPTA intensities of pulsed and continuous-wave ultrasound are compared, the appropriate time to be used is
  a. the total exposure time
  b. the sound-on time
7.4.3 When SPTP intensity of pulsed ultrasound is compared with SPTA intensity of continuous-wave ultrasound, the appropriate time to be used is
  a. the total exposure time
  b. the sound-on time

7.4.4 The sound-on time is the total time multiplied by
   a. beam uniformity ratio
   b. pulse repetition frequency
   c. doppler shift
   d. reflection coefficient
   e. duty factor

7.5
Safety

For consideration of the safety of diagnostic ultrasound, an attempt must be made to relate knowledge of bioeffects to the clinical situation (Fig. 7.25). There are three questions that arise when an attempt is made to accomplish this:

1. Do any of the bioeffects that have occurred under experimental conditions constitute a hazard to a human in the clinical setting?
2. Are the acoustic parameters at the site of the bioeffect in experimental animals comparable to those at the appropriate site of concern in the human body during diagnosis?
3. Do the continuous-wave conditions of most experimental studies provide any useful information for the pulsed ultrasound of clinical diagnosis?

These questions remain largely unanswered. As there is no satisfying response to question 1, an attempt must be made to determine if *any* bioeffects observed in experimental animals are likely to occur clinically. This brings us to the difficulties of questions 2 and 3. The response to question 2 is that in human applications of ultrasound, the organs of concern are normally farther from the sound source (a longer attenuating sound path is involved). Also, a smaller organ volume fraction is exposed because the organs are larger than those of the experimental animals. Experimental studies are normally done with a stationary sound beam, whereas diagnostic studies usually involve scanning. These considerations may provide some (unknown) safety factors for the diagnostic situation. Concerning question 3, it is not known whether or not short diagnostic pulses of low duty factor can produce bioeffects under clinical conditions and whether or not repair could occur between pulses.

Because a complete knowledge of bioeffects is unavailable, a conservative approach to safety considerations must be taken. Use diagnostic

Figure 7.25. Relating bioeffects information to risk determination. Unanswered questions limit our ability to determine the relationship thoroughly.

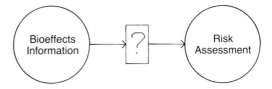

ultrasound in an appropriate manner when benefit is expected from the procedure. What constitutes "appropriate manner"? The following is quoted from an AIUM brochure on the subject[26]:

Diagnostic ultrasound has proven to be a valuable tool in medical practice and should be used without hesitation, with appropriate equipment and procedures, when medical benefit is expected. An excellent safety record exists in that after decades of clinical use there is no known instance of human injury due to diagnostic ultrasound.

Users should be aware of the factors related to ultrasonic exposure levels and should give serious consideration to intensity data when comparing various instruments. Other factors such as imaging quality, convenience, etc., are important, but if various instruments are equivalent in these aspects, the instrument with the lowest intensity levels should be favored. Increasing numbers of manufacturers are supplying intensity data for their equipment. The AIUM encourages the release of these data. Any manufacturer displaying the AIUM Manufacturer's Commendation Award for a specified model has satisfied AIUM requirements for determining exposure data for that model and for making the information publicly available.

It is important that users understand how they can minimize exposures in obtaining needed diagnostic information. Obviously, the shorter the examination, the less is the total exposure to the patient. In some equipment, controls are available which adjust the excitation of the transducer and change the emitted peak intensity or pulse repetition frequency. Different types of transducers can also exhibit different emitted intensity levels.

In assessing risk, overly simplistic attitudes should be avoided. The SPTA intensity of 100 mW/cm^2 should not be treated as a magic number. Levels under

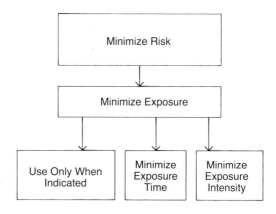

Figure 7.26. Minimize risk by minimizing exposure.

this value do not guarantee "perfect" safety, and levels above this value may well be appropriate if they are needed to yield diagnostic information. In choosing procedures and equipment, the obligation is always present to balance benefit against risk.

In short, we should minimize (unknown, but potentially non-zero) risk by minimizing exposure (Fig. 7.26).

The AIUM issued the following 1987 statements regarding epidemiology:

Epidemiology
1. Widespread clinical use over 25 years has not established any adverse effect arising from exposure to diagnostic ultrasound.
2. Randomized clinical studies are the most rigorous method for assessing potential adverse effects of diagnostic ultrasound. Studies using this methodology show no evidence of an effect on birthweight in humans.*
3. Other epidemiologic studies have shown no causal association of diagnostic ultrasound with any of the adverse fetal outcomes studied.*

---

*The acoustic exposure levels in these studies may not be representative of the full range of current fetal exposures.

The AIUM has issued two statements[26] (March and October 1983, revised March 1988) dealing with safety of diagnostic ultrasound in clinical care, education, and research:

Statement on Clinical Safety
Diagnostic ultrasound has been in use since the late 1950s. Given its known benefits and recognized efficacy for medical diagnosis, including use during human pregnancy, the American Institute of Ultrasound in Medicine herein addresses the clinical safety of such use:

No confirmed biological effects on patients or instrument operators caused by exposures at intensities typical of present diagnostic instruments have ever been reported. Although the possibility exists that such biological effects may be identified in the future, current data indicate that the benefits to patients of the prudent use of diagnostic ultrasound outweigh the risks, if any, that may be present.

Safety Statement for Training and Research
Diagnostic ultrasound has been in use since the late 1950s. No confirmed adverse biologic effects on patients or instrument operators caused by exposure at intensities and exposure conditions typical of present diagnostic instrument and examination practices have ever been reported. Experience from normal diagnostic practice may or may not be relevant to extended exposure times and altered exposure conditions. At this time, no hazard has been identified that would preclude the prudent and conservative use of diagnostic ultrasound in education and research.

Exercises

7.5.1 The available epidemiologic data are sufficient to make a final judgment on the safety of diagnostic ultrasound. True or false?
7.5.2 Exposure is minimized by using diagnostic ultrasound
   a. only when indicated
   b. with minimum intensity
   c. with minimum time
   d. all of the above
   e. none of the above

7.6
Review

The 100-mm test object provides a means of measuring axial and lateral resolution, range and registration accuracy, dead zone, compensation, sensitivity, and dynamic range of diagnostic instruments. Beam profilers measure characteristics of beams produced by transducers. Hydrophones are used to measure the acoustic output of diagnostic instruments.

The AIUM has stated that there have been no independently confirmed significant bioeffects in mammalian tissues exposed to SPTA intensities below 100 mW/cm^2. This indicates that with some instruments that operate at the higher intensities, it may be possible to produce some bioeffects in small animals. Whether or not they can occur in humans is unknown. Because there is limited specific knowledge, the conservative approach is taken: use diagnostic ultrasound with minimum exposure when benefit is expected from the procedure.

Definitions of terms discussed in this chapter are listed below:

Beam profiler. A device that plots three-dimensional reflection amplitude information.

Cavitation. Production and behavior of bubbles in sound.

Dead zone. Region close to the transducer in which imaging cannot be performed.

Hydrophone. A small transducer element mounted on the end of a narrow tube.

Phantom. Tissue-equivalent device that has some characteristics representative of tissues (e.g., scattering or attenuation properties).

Test object. A device designed to measure some characteristic of an imaging system without having tissue-like properties.

Exercises

7.6.1 Match these devices or phenomena with what they measure (answers may be used more than once):
   a. beam profiler: _____
   b. 100-mm test object:

   _____, _____
   c. hydrophone: _____,

   _____
   1. diagnostic instrument imaging performance
   2. transducer beam characteristics
   3. diagnostic instrument acoustic output

7.6.2 Match the following with the components about which they usually provide information:
   a. hydrophone: _____
   b. beam profiler: _____
   c. 100-mm test object: _____
   1. diagnostic instrument as a whole
   2. pulser and transducer
   3. transducer
   4. transducer and receiver
   5. receiver and display

7.6.3 There is no possible hazard involved in the diagnostic use of ultrasound. True or false?

7.6.4 Ultrasound should not be used as a diagnostic tool because of the bioeffects it can produce. True or false?

7.6.5 No independently confirmed significant bioeffects in mammalian tissues have been reported at intensities below

   a. 10 W/cm^2 SPTP

   b. 100 mW/cm^2 SPTA

   c. 10 mW/cm^2 SPTA

   d. 10 mW/cm^2 SATA

   e. 1 mW/cm^2 SATP

7.6.6 Is there any knowledge of what types of injuries or risks occur with diagnostic ultrasound in patients, and under what conditions? Yes or no?

7.6.7 Is there any knowledge of any bioeffects that ultrasound produces in small animals under experimental conditions? Yes or no?

Chapter 8

Summary

By sending short pulses of ultrasound into the body and using reflected and scattered sound received from tissue interfaces and from within tissues to produce images of internal structures, ultrasound is used as a medical diagnostic tool. Ultrasound is a wave of traveling acoustic variables described by frequency, period, wavelength, propagation speed, amplitude, intensity, and attenuation.

Pulsed ultrasound is used in ultrasound imaging. It is described, additionally, by pulse repetition frequency and period, pulse duration, duty factor, and spatial pulse length. Pulses contain a range of frequencies described by bandwidth and Q factor. Diagnostic ultrasound commonly uses frequencies from 2 to 10 MHz, SPTA intensities from 0.01 to 200 mW/cm^2, pulse repetition frequencies from 0.5 to 4 kHz, duty factors from 0.001 to 0.003, and pulses of from 2 to 3 cycles. Soft-tissue propagation speed is 1.54 mm/μs, and the attenuation coefficient is 0.5 dB/cm for each MHz of frequency.

For *perpendicular incidence* at boundaries, reflections are produced if media impedances (density x propagation speed) are different. For *oblique incidence*, refraction occurs if media propagation speeds are different. Scattering occurs at rough boundaries and within heterogeneous media. Scattering strength increases with increasing frequency. A doppler shift is produced if a reflector or scatterer is moving. The distance to reflectors is determined by round-trip travel time.

Transducers convert electric energy to ultrasound energy and vice versa by piezoelectricity. Axial resolution is equal to one half the spatial pulse length, which can be reduced by damping or increasing frequency (improving resolution). Lateral resolution is equal to beam diameter, which can be reduced by focusing (improving resolution). These
232

resolutions (with focusing) are approximately 1 mm. Disc transducers produce sound beams with near and far zones. Focusing can only be accomplished in the near zone of the comparable unfocused transducer. Arrays can scan, steer, and shape beams repeatedly, permitting dynamic imaging. Dynamic imaging can also be accomplished with mechanically driven single-element transducers or mirrors.

Pulse-echo systems use the amplitude, direction, and arrival time of reflections to produce A, B, or M mode displays. Imaging systems consist of pulser, transducer, receiver, memory, and display. Pulsers set the pulse repetition frequency, which determines maximum unambiguous imaging depth. Receivers amplify, compensate, compress, and demodulate echo voltage pulses. Scan converters store gray-scale image information and permit display on a television monitor. They are of two types—analog and digital. The number of bits per pixel in a digital memory determines the contrast resolution. Dynamic imaging instruments display a rapid sequence of static pictures. Doppler instruments use the doppler shift of reflections to produce audible sound or images characteristic of motion. Pulsed doppler instruments obtain range information. Spectral analysis provides a quantitative measure of doppler information. Color-flow instruments display two-dimensional real-time representations of flow.

Display artifacts include resolution, texture, section thickness, reverberation, refraction, side and grating lobes, multipath, mirror image, shadowing, enhancement, speed error, and range ambiguity.

Imaging performance is measured with test objects and tissue equivalent (TE) phantoms. Acoustic output is measured with hydrophones. Beam profilers, test objects, and hydrophones measure transducer beam characteristics. Spectrum analyzers measure frequency content of ultrasound pulses.

There have been no independently confirmed significant bioeffects in mammalian tissues exposed to SPTA intensities below 100 mW/cm^2. Current data indicate that the benefits to patients of the prudent use of diagnostic ultrasound outweigh any potential risk.

Exercises

8.1 Increasing the frequency
   a. improves the resolution
   b. increases the half-intensity depth
   c. increases refraction
   d. both a and b
   e. both a and c

8.2 Increasing the pulse repetition frequency
   a. improves resolution
   b. increases maximum depth imaged unambiguously
   c. decreases maximum depth imaged unambiguously
   d. both a and b
   e. both a and c

8.3 Increasing the intensity produced by the transducer
   a. is accomplished by increasing the pulser voltage
   b. increases the sensitivity of the system
   c. increases the probability of bioeffects
   d. all of the above
   e. none of the above

8.4 Increasing the spatial pulse length
   a. is accomplished by transducer damping
   b. is accompanied by decreased pulse duration
   c. improves the axial resolution
   d. all of the above
   e. none of the above

8.5 Dynamic imaging is made possible by
   a. scan converters
   b. mechanically driven transducers
   c. gray-scale display
   d. arrays
   e. both b and d

8.6 The 100-mm test object measures
   a. resolution
   b. pulse duration
   c. SATA intensity
   d. wavelength
   e. all of the above

8.7 The following measure acoustic output:
   a. hydrophone
   b. scan converter
   c. 100-mm test object
   d. all of the above
   e. none of the above

8.8 Ultrasound bioeffects
   a. do not occur
   b. do not occur with diagnostic instruments
   c. are not confirmed below $100 \ mW/cm^2$ SPTA
   d. both b and c
   e. none of the above

8.9 The diagnostic ultrasound frequency range is

a. 2 to 10 mHz
b. 2 to 10 kHz
c. 2 to 10 MHz
d. 3 to 15 kHz
e. none of the above

8.10 Small transducers always produce smaller beam diameters. True or false?

8.11 No reflection occurs if media impedances are equal. True or false?

8.12 No refraction occurs if media impedances are equal. True or false?

8.13 Gray-scale display is made possible by
a. array transducers
b. cathode ray storage tubes
c. scan converters
d. both b and c
e. all of the above

8.14 Attenuation is corrected for by
a. demodulation
b. desegregation
c. decompression
d. compensation

8.15 Vertical deflections of the display spot are produced by reflections in
a. the B mode
b. the doppler mode
c. the M mode
d. the a la mode
e. none of the above

8.16 The doppler effect for a scatterer moving toward the transducer causes scattered sound (compared with the incident sound) received by the transducer to have _____.
a. increased intensity
b. decreased intensity
c. increased impedance
d. increased frequency
e. decreased impedance

8.17 An ultrasound instrument that could represent 64 shades of gray would require an eight-bit memory. True or false?

8.18 Continuous-wave sound is used in _____.
a. all imaging instruments
b. some imaging instruments
c. all doppler instruments
d. some doppler instruments
e. none of the above

8.19 What is the transmitted intensity if the incident intensity is 1 and
the impedances are 1.00 and 2.64?
a. 0.2
b. 0.4
c. 0.6
d. 0.8
e. 1.0

8.20 Match the following (answers may be used more than once):
a. A mode: _____, _____,   1. one-dimensional (spatial)
_____   2. two-dimensional (spatial)
b. B scan: _____, _____, _____   3. real-time
c. M mode: _____, _____,   4. deflection
_____   5. brightness

8.21 An advantage of continuous-wave doppler instruments is that they
have _____.
a. no aliasing
b. depth information and selectivity
c. bidirectional information
d. amplitude information
e. all of the above

8.22 An advantage of pulsed doppler instruments is that they have

_____.
a. no aliasing
b. depth information
c. bidirectional information
d. amplitude information
e. all of the above

8.23 A digital memory with one bit per pixel would have a
_____ display.
a. bidirectional
b. biscattering
c. bistable

8.24 If a transducer element 19 mm in diameter is focused to produce a
minimum beam diameter of 2 mm, the intensity at the focus is approximately _____ times the intensity at the transducer.
a. 2
b. 3
c. 19
d. 100
e. 500

8.25 The largest number that can be stored in a pixel of a seven-bit
digital memory is _____.
a. 16
b. 32

c. 127
d. 255
e. 256

8.26 Digital calipers provide a measurement of distance between
_____.
a. potentiometers
b. bits
c. optical encoders
d. pixels
e. all of the above

8.27 Which of the following produce(s) a sector-scan format?
a. rotating mechanic real-time transducer
b. oscillating mechanical real-time transducer
c. phased array
d. oscillating mirror
e. all of the above

8.28 A digital imaging instrument divides the cross-sectional image into
_____.
a. frequencies
b. bits
c. pixels
d. binaries
e. wavelengths

8.29 Digital scan converters have better _____ than analog
scan converters.
a. spatial resolution
b. gray-scale resolution
c. sensitivity
d. reliability
e. efficiency

8.30 The binary number 10111 is equal to the decimal number
_____.
a. 10
b. 16
c. 20
d. 23
e. 111

8.31 The axial resolution for a two-cycle pulse of 5 MHz in tissue is _____
mm.
a. 0.1
b. 0.2
c. 0.3
d. 0.4
e. 0.5

8.32 The best lateral resolution for an unfocused 13-mm transducer element is _____ mm.
   a. 2.5
   b. 4.5
   c. 6.5
   d. 815
   e. 13

8.33 If the frequency of the element in Exercise 8.32 is 3.5 MHz, the near-zone length is _____ cm.
   a. 5
   b. 10
   c. 15
   d. 20
   e. 25

8.34 Can the element of Exercise 8.33 be focused at 5 cm? Yes or no?

8.35 If pulse repetition frequency is increased, the SPTA intensity is _____.
   a. increased
   b. unchanged
   c. decreased
   d. eliminated
   e. none of the above

8.36 If the thickness of a transducer element is decreased, the frequency is _____.
   a. increased
   b. unchanged
   c. decreased
   d. intensified
   e. none of the above

8.37 In Exercise 8.36, the near-zone length is _____.
   a. increased
   b. unchanged
   c. decreased
   d. intensified
   e. none of the above

8.38 With increased damping, which of the following is increased?
   a. bandwidth
   b. pulse duration
   c. spatial pulse length
   d. Q factor
   e. all of the above

8.39 As frequency is increased, which of the following are decreased?
   a. propagation speed

b. half-intensity depth
c. imaging depth
d. more than one of the above
e. none of the above

8.40 If a static image is produced by a 3-s scan, there will be approximately _____ scan lines in the image.
a. 3
b. 100
c. 300
d. 3000
e. 30,000

8.41 If linear preprocessing is used and the echo dynamic range is 40 dB, a 20-dB echo will be assigned the number _____ in a six-bit memory.
a. 0
b. 16
c. 32
d. 48
e. 64

8.42 If linear postprocessing is used, a stored 48 in a six-bit memory will produce _____ per cent brightness on the display.
a. 0
b. 15
c. 50
d. 75
e. 100

8.43 A five-bit memory can store which of the following numbers?
a. 64
b. 32
c. 31
d. 55
e. all of the above

8.44 Television monitors produce _____ frames per second.
a. 10
b. 24
c. 30
d. 60
e. none of the above

8.45 Duplex doppler instruments include _____.
a. pulsed doppler
b. continuous wave doppler
c. static imaging
d. dynamic imaging
e. more than one of the above

8.46 Match the following modes of display with the information that can be obtained:

a. A mode: _____, _____   1. reflector motion
b. M mode: _____, _____   2. reflector distance
c. static B scan: _____, _____   3. reflector shape
d. dynamic B scan: _____,   4. reflector density
_____, _____

8.47 If the doppler shifts from normal and from stenotic carotid arteries are 4 kHz and 10 kHz, respectively, for which will there be a problem with a pulse repetition frequency of 7 kHz?

a. normal
b. stenotic
c. both
d. neither

8.48 Compensation (swept gain) makes up for the fact that reflections from deeper reflectors arrive at the transducer later. True or false?

8.49 Which of the following affects gray-scale resolution?

a. number of pixels
b. number of bits per pixel
c. pulse duration
d. frequency
e. focusing

8.50 Which of the following requires a phased array as a receiving transducer?

a. dynamic range
b. dynamic imaging
c. dynamic focusing
d. none of the above

8.51 Across:

1. Referring to sound
2. Abbreviation for cosine
3. Not perpendicular to a boundary
4. Occurs at boundaries with perpendicular incidence
5. Material through which sound is passing
6. Pulsed doppler requires _____ the receiver
7. The duty _____ is sound-on fraction
8. Beam diameter decreases in the _____ zone
9. Intensity is power divided by _____
10. Reflector motion produces a doppler _____
11. Sound of frequency 20 kHz and higher
12. Parallel to sound direction
13. Maximum variation of an acoustic variable
14. Abbreviation for continuous wave

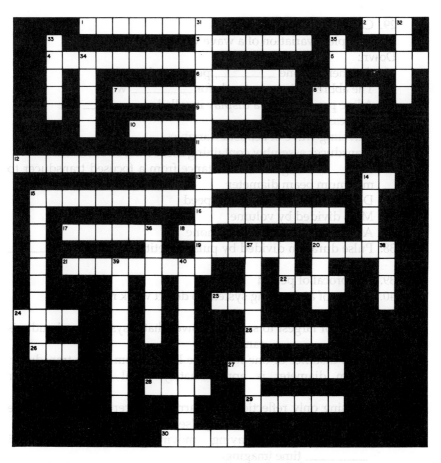

15. Attenuation _____ is given in decibels per centimeter
16. Power divided by area
17. Reciprocal of frequency
18. The range equation gives distance _____ a reflector
19. Perpendicular to a boundary
20. Displacement divided by time
21. Propagation speed depends on density and _____
22. _____ scale displays several values of spot brightness
23. Beam diameter increases in the _____ zone
24. Force times displacement
25. Axial resolution depends on spatial _____ length
26. Abbreviation for sine
27. Reflected frequency minus incident frequency equals _____ shift
28. A traveling variation

29. Capability for doing work
30. Complete variation of a wave variable
Down:
14. One hertz is one _____ per second
15. The abbreviation cw stands for _____ wave
20. A line produced on a display is called a _____ line
31. (A message for you)
32. Traveling wave of acoustic variables
33. Transducer assembly containing more than one element
34. _____ length is the distance from a focused transducer to minimum beam diameter
35. Density times propagation speed
36. Mass divided by volume
37. Another name for a hydrophone
38. Pulse duration divided by pulse repetition period is _____ factor
39. Reciprocal of period
40. Ability of an imaging system to detect weak reflections

8.52 Across:
1. Ratio of largest to smallest power that a system can handle is called _____ range.
2. At a distance of one near-zone length from a disc transducer, beam diameter is approximately equal to disc diameter divided by _____.
3. Passing only reflections that arrive at a certain time after the transducer has produced a pulse is called _____.
4. Continuously displaying moving structures is called _____ time imaging.
5. Increasing small voltages to larger ones.
6. The speed with which a wave moves through a medium is called _____ speed.
7. The region of a sound beam where beam diameter increases with distance from the transducer is called the _____ zone.
8. Another word for a reflection.
9. Acoustic means having to do with _____.
10. If propagation speeds of two media are equal, incidence angle equals _____ angle.
11. A device that stores a gray-scale image and allows it to be displayed on a television monitor is called a scan _____.
12. Conversion of sound to heat.
13. Power divided by area.
14. An echo-free region on a display is called _____.

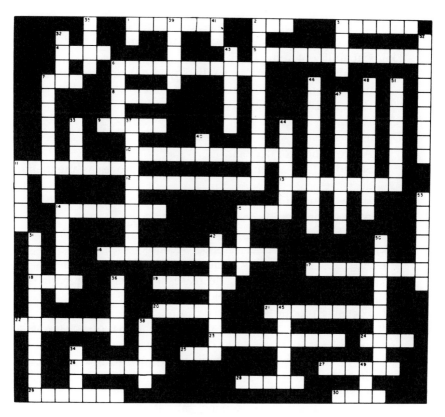

15. The fraction of time that pulsed ultrasound is actually on is called _____ factor.

16. The AIUM statement on bioeffects says that there have been no _____ confirmed significant bioeffects below 100 mW/cm^2.

17. Density multiplied by sound propagation speed.

18. Displaying several values of spot brightness is carried out on a _____ scale.

19. If no reflection occurs at a boundary, this always means that media impedances are equal in the case of _____ incidence.

20. A few cycles of ultrasound may be called an ultrasound _____.

21. Maximum variation of an acoustic variable or voltage.

22. Reverberations are also called _____ reflections.

23. A device that converts energy from one form to another.

24. Prefix meaning 1000.

25. Abbreviation for megahertz.

26. _____ incidence is when the sound direction is not per-
    pendicular to the boundary of the medium.
27. Capability of doing work.
28. Number of complete scans displayed per unit time in a real-
    time system is called the _____ rate.
29. Perpendicular to the direction of sound travel.
30. A unit for impedance.

Down:

1. Abbreviation for decibel.
2. Sound _____ through a medium improves as attenuation
   decreases.
3. Ratio of output to input electrical power for an amplifier.
6. A Greek prefix meaning pressure.
7. Number of cycles per unit time.
11. One hertz is one _____ per second.
14. An _____ array is made up of ring-shaped elements.
15. Half-intensity _____ decreases with increasing frequency.
31. Along the direction of sound travel (axial).
32. Focusing produces decreased beam _____.
33. A sound _____ is a traveling variation of acoustic
    variables.
34. Most two-dimensional imaging is done with B _____
    displays.
35. To sweep a sound beam to produce an image.
36. Rate at which work is done; rate at which energy is trans-
    ferred.
37. Sound of frequency greater than 20 kHz.
38. Concentrate the sound beam into a smaller area.
39. A transducer _____ is an assembly containing more than
    one transducer element.
40. Abbreviation for millimeter.
41. Abbreviation for continuous wave.
42. Frequency unit.
43. A _____ array is made up of rectangular elements in a
    line.
44. Propagation speed increases with decreasing _____.
45. Material through which a wave travels.
46. Decrease of amplitude and intensity as a wave travels through
    a medium.
47. Length of space over which a cycle occurs.
48. Change of sound direction on passing from one medium to
    another.
49. A cathode _____ tube is a common display device.

50. Diffusion or redirection of sound in several directions.
51. Speed, with direction of motion specified.
52. Perpendicular _____ occurs when sound direction is perpendicular to the boundary of the medium.
53. The _____ effect is a frequency change of reflected sound wave due to reflector motion.

Exercise 8.52 from Kremkau, F.W.: Crossword puzzle. Med. Ultrasound, 4:38, 1980. Reprinted by permission of John Wiley & Sons, Inc.

8.53 Identify the physical terms, the common measurement units for which are given.

Across:
1. joule
2. microsecond
3. rayl
4. joule
5. decibel
6. kelvin
7. millimeter
8. gram
9. milliliter
10. hertz

Down:
5. radian
11. meter/second
12. newton/meter^2
13. watt
14. newton
15. decibel
16. meter/second^2
17. centimeter^2
18. watt/centimeter^2
19. second
20. gram/milliliter

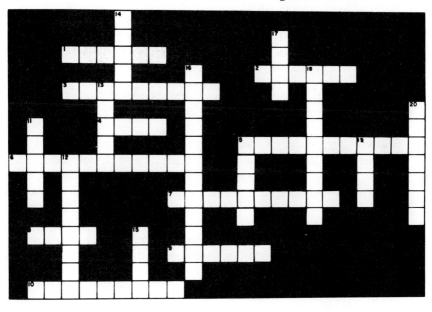

Exercise 8.53 from Kremkau, F.W.: Ultrapuzzles. Reflections 6:85, 1980. Reprinted by permission of the American Institute of Ultrasound in Medicine.

8.54 In the following review, blanks need to be filled in. In the figure, begin at the upper left and draw a line to one letter at a time in any direction (horizontal, vertical, or diagonal) to spell out the words for the blanks. All letters are used in a continuous line. Do not cross over your line. Use each letter only once. The words should be found in the same order as they are needed for the blanks.

Ultrasound is a _____ of traveling _____ variables.

START

W								
A	F	R	E	Q	U	S	P	O	P
V	C	I	T	S	E	E	R	A	E
E	A	C	O	U	N	I	G	T	R
E	E	P	S	N	C	A	A	T	I
D	A	T	T	O	T	S	C	N	G
A	U	N	E	I	Z	T	R	E	T
T	I	O	N	M	E	G	A	H	R
R	O	M	E	R	E	D	S	N	A
Y	S	P	M	S	C	U	U	E	N
D	I	L	A	Y	S	E	Q	C	E

END

Pulsed ultrasound is commonly used in ultrasound imaging. Pulses contain a range of _____. Soft tissue _____ _____ is 1.54 mm/µs and the _____ coefficient is 1 dB/cm for each _____ of frequency. _____ occurs at rough boundaries and within heterogeneous media. _____ convert electrical energy to ultrasound energy and vice versa. Imaging systems consist of pulser, transducer, receiver, _____, and _____. Dynamic imaging instruments display a rapid ____ of static pictures.

8.55 Propagation speed increases with increasing

    a. stiffness
    b. density
    c. absorption
    d. attenuation
    e. both a and b

8.56 Reflections are produced by changes in

    a. stiffness
    b. density
    c. absorption
    d. attenuation
    e. both a and b

8.57 If no reflection occurs at a boundary, this always means that media impedances are equal in the case of

    a. perpendicular incidence
    b. oblique incidence
    c. refraction
    d. both a and b
    e. both b and c

8.58 If the propagation speeds in two media are equal, the refraction equation states that the incidence angle equals the

    a. reflection angle
    b. transmission angle
    c. doppler angle
    d. both a and b
    e. both b and c

8.59 At a distance of one near-zone length from a disc transducer, the beam diameter is equal to the disc diameter divided by

    a. one
    b. two
    c. three
    d. π
    e. one fourth

8.60 Velocity is _____.

    a. speed
    b. direction
    c. acceleration
    d. a and b
    e. all of the above

8.61 Decibels are _____ ratio units.
   a. amplitude
   b. power
   c. neper
   d. more than one of the above
   e. all of the above

8.62 Which of the following can be real-time? (More than one correct answer)
   a. A mode
   b. B mode
   c. B scan
   d. M mode
   e. doppler

8.63 A characteristic of an AIUM 100-mm test object that may produce incorrect results is
   a. weight of the liquid
   b. age of the liquid
   c. sound speed in the liquid
   d. temperature of the rods
   e. none of the above

8.64 The following test(s) can be performed using the AIUM 100-mm test object
   a. dead zone
   b. resolution
   c. registration accuracy
   d. range accuracy
   e. all of the above

8.65 If all six rods of the central groups in an AIUM 100-mm test object appear separately on a display of the object, the axial resolution is
   a. 1 mm
   b. 2 mm
   c. 3 mm
   d. 4 mm
   e. 5 mm

8.66 Which of the following produce(s) a sector scan format?
   a. rotating mechanical real-time transducer
   b. oscillating mechanical real-time transducer
   c. phased array
   d. linear switched array
   e. more than one of the above

8.67 Which of the following produce(s) a rectangular scan format?
  a. rotating mechanical real-time transducer
  b. oscillating mechanical real-time transducer
  c. phased array
  d. linear switched array
  e. more than one of the above

8.68 Gray-scale displays present brightness corresponding to echo
  a. frequency
  b. amplitude
  c. bandwidth
  d. impedance
  e. more than one of the above

8.69 If approximately 100 different gray levels can be distinguished by a human observer, how may bits per pixel would be a good choice for an ultrasound memory?
  a. 4
  b. 6
  c. 8
  d. 10
  e. 12

8.70 Which of the following memories will have sufficient contrast resolution to distinguish adjacent 25 and 26 dB echoes within a 0 to 40 dB dynamic range assuming straight line pre- and postprocessing characteristics?
  a. 5 bit
  b. 6 bit
  c. 7 bit
  d. b and c
  e. all of the above

8.71 A digital scan converter stores _____ corresponding to echo amplitudes.
  a. numbers
  b. electrical charges
  c. lines
  d. frames
  e. none of the above

8.72 Intensity of returning echoes changes with angle in doppler flow measurements (true or false)?

8.73 Intensity of returning echoes changes with flow speed in doppler ultrasound (true or false)?

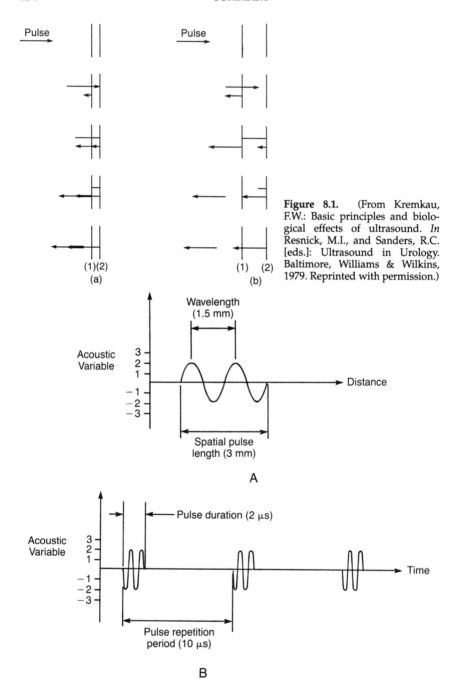

Figure 8.1. (From Kremkau, F.W.: Basic principles and biological effects of ultrasound. *In* Resnick, M.I., and Sanders, R.C. [eds.]: Ultrasound in Urology. Baltimore, Williams & Wilkins, 1979. Reprinted with permission.)

Figure 8.2. (From Kremkau, F.W.: Basic principles and biological effects of ultrasound. *In* Resnick, M.I., and Sanders, R.C. [eds.]: Ultrasound in Urology. Baltimore, Williams & Wilkins, 1979. Reprinted with permission.)

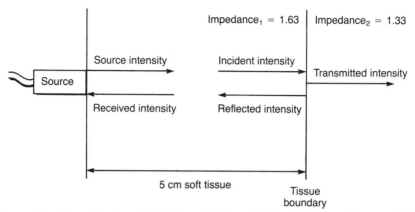

Figure 8.3 (From Kremkau, F.W.: Basic principles and biological effects of ultrasound. *In* Resnick, M.I., and Sanders, R.C. [eds.]: Ultrasound in Urology. Baltimore, Williams & Wilkins, 1979. Reprinted with permission.)

8.74 Figure 8.1 describes which resolution?
  a. axial
  b. lateral
  c. contrast
  d. detail
  e. a and d
8.75 In which part of Figure 8.1 (a or b) are the two reflectors resolved?
8.76 In Figure 8.2, give the following:
  a. number of cycles in a pulse
  b. amplitude
  c. wavelength
  d. spatial pulse length
  e. pulse repetition period
  f. pulse repetition frequency
  g. pulse duration
  h. period
  i. frequency
  j. duty factor
  k. propagation speed
8.77 In Figure 8.3, if the frequency is 4 MHz, the attenuation from the source to the tissue boundary is _____ dB. If the intensity emitted by the source (transducer) is 10 mW/cm^2, the intensity arriving at the boundary (incident intensity) is _____ mW/cm^2. The intensity reflection coefficient at the boundary is _____. The reflected intensity is _____ mW/cm^2 and the received intensity at the source is _____ mW/cm^2.

Propagation Speed₁   Propagation Speed₂

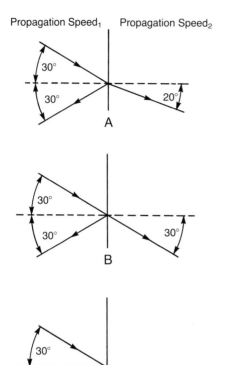

Figure 8.4. (From Kremkau, F.W.: Basic principles and biological effects of ultrasound. *In* Resnick, M.I., and Sanders, R.C. [eds.]: Ultrasound in Urology. Baltimore, Williams & Wilkins, 1979. Reprinted with permission.)

8.78 In which part of Figure 8.4 (a, b, c) is speed (2) greater than speed (1); is speed (2) less than speed (1); is speed (2) equal to speed (1); is there no refraction?

8.79 Figure 8.5 shows that a higher frequency yields a (longer, shorter) near-zone length and that a larger transducer produces a (longer, shorter) near-zone length. By curving them, which of these transducers (a, b, c, d) can be focused at 25 cm; at 15 cm; at 4 cm?

8.80 In Figure 8.6, the wave type is (continuous-wave, pulsed), if the lower portion of the figure represents 4 ms later than the upper portion, the propagation speed is _____ mm/μs, the wavelength for 1 MHz frequency is _____ mm, and the spatial pulse length is _____ mm.

8.81 In Figure 8.7, the frequency is _____ MHz, the period is _____ μs, the amplitude is _____ units, the wave type is (continous-wave or pulsed), and for soft tissue the wavelength is _____ mm.

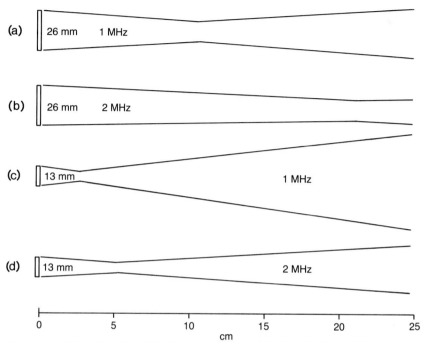

Figure 8.5. (From Kremkau, F.W.: Basic principles and biological effects of ultrasound. *In* Resnick, M.I., and Sanders, R.C. [eds.]: Ultrasound in Urology. Baltimore, Williams & Wilkins, 1979. Reprinted with permission.)

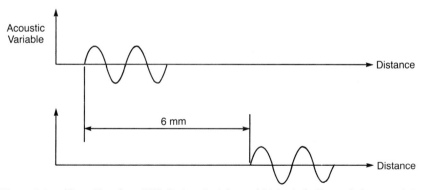

Figure 8.6. (From Kremkau, F.W.: Basic principles and biological effects of ultrasound. *In* Resnick, M.I., and Sanders, R.C. [eds.]: Ultrasound in Urology. Baltimore, Williams & Wilkins, 1979. Reprinted with permission.)

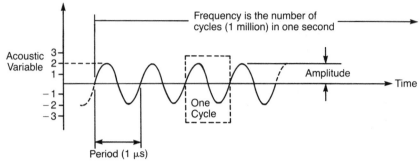

Figure 8.7 (From Kremkau, F.W.: Basic principles and biological effects of ultrasound. *In* Resnick, M.I., and Sanders, R.C. [eds.]: Ultrasound in Urology. Baltimore, Williams & Wilkins, 1979. Reprinted with permission.)

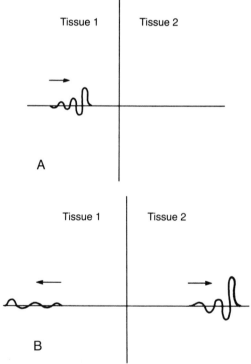

Figure 8.8. (From Kremkau, F.W.: Ultrasound instrumentation: Physical principles. *In* Callen, P.W. [ed.]: Ultrasonography in Obstetrics and Gynecology. Philadelphia, W.B. Saunders Co., 1982. Reprinted with permission.)

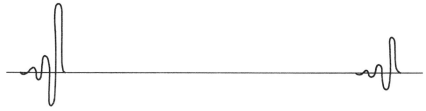

Figure 8.9. (From Kremkau, F.W.: Ultrasound instrumentation: Physical principles. *In* Callen, P.W. [ed.]: Ultrasonography in Obstetrics and Gynecology. Philadelphia, W.B. Saunders Co., 1982. Reprinted with permission.)

8.82 In Figure 8.8, which of the following have occurred?
  a. reflection
  b. refraction
  c. transmission
  d. a and b
  e. a and c

8.83 In Figure 8.9, as the pulse travels to the right, the amplitude decreases. This is called _____. If the amplitude at the right is one half the amplitude at the left, the attenuation is _____ dB. If the distance from left to right is 3 cm, the attenuation coefficient is _____ dB/cm. If the travel were in soft tissue, the frequency of the pulse would be approximately _____ MHz.

8.84 In Figure 8.10, which is the higher frequency pulse?
  a. a
  b. b
  c. neither

8.85 In Figure 8.10, which pulse travels faster?
  a. a
  b. b
  c. neither

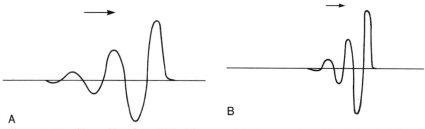

A   B

Figure 8.10 (From Kremkau, F.W.: Ultrasound instrumentation: Physical principles. *In* Callen, P.W. [ed.]: Ultrasonography in Obstetrics and Gynecology. Philadelphia, W.B. Saunders Co., 1982. Reprinted with permission.)

8.86 In Figure 8.10, which pulse travels farther (experiences less attenuation)?
   a. a
   b. b
   c. neither
8.87 In Figure 8.10, which pulse has the better axial resolution?
   a. a
   b. b
   c. neither
8.88 In Figure 8.10, which pulse has the greater amplitude?
   a. a
   b. b
   c. neither
8.89 As frequency increases, which of the following (more than one) decrease?
   a. period
   b. wavelength
   c. propagation speed
   d. amplitude
   e. intensity
   f. attenuation coefficient
   g. half-intensity depth
   h. reflection coefficient
   i. transmission coefficient
   j. refraction
   k. pulse duration
   l. spatial pulse length
   m. pulse repetition frequency
   n. pulse repetition period
   o. duty factor
   p. near-zone length
   q. imaging depth
   r. axial resolution
   s. impedance
8.90 This textbook is
   a. enjoyable
   b. profitable
   c. relevant
   d. well done
   e. complete
   f. accurate
   g. concise
   h. stimulating

i. simple
j. clear
k. error-freee
m. omission-free
o. helpful
p. great
q. perfect
r. all of the above

Glossary

The terms defined here are listed at the end of the chapter in which they are discussed.

A mode. Mode of operation in which the display records a vertical spot deflection for each pulse delivered from the receiver.

Absorption. Conversion of sound to heat.

Acceleration. Change in velocity divided by time over which the change occurs.

Acoustic. Having to do with sound.

Acoustic propagation properties. Characteristics of a medium that affect the propagation of sound through it.

Acoustic variables. Pressure, density, temperature, and particle motion—things that are functions of space and time in a sound wave.

Aliasing. Improper doppler shift information from a pulsed doppler instrument when true doppler shift exceeds half the pulse repetition frequency.

Amplification. Increasing small voltages to larger ones.

Amplifier. A device that accomplishes amplification.

Amplitude. Maximum variation of an acoustic variable or voltage.

Analog. Related to a procedure or system in which data are represented by continuously variable physical quantities (e.g., electrical charge).

Annular array. Array made up of ring-shaped elements arranged concentrically.

Array. Transducer array.

Attenuation. Decrease in amplitude and intensity as a wave travels through a medium.

Attenuation coefficient. Attenuation per unit length of wave travel.

Autocorrelation. A rapid technique for obtaining mean doppler shift frequency. This technique is used in color-flow instruments.

Axial. In the direction of the transducer axis (sound-travel direction).

Axial resolution. Minimum reflector separation along the sound path required for separate reflections to be produced.

B mode. Mode of operation in which the display records a spot brightening for each echo pulse delivered from the receiver.

B scan. A brightness image that represents a cross section of the object through the scanning plane.

Backscatter. Sound scattered back in the direction from which it originally came.

Bandwidth. Range of frequencies contained in an ultrasound pulse.

Beam area. Cross-sectional area of a sound beam.

Beam profiler. A device that plots three-dimensional reflection amplitude information.

Beam uniformity ratio. Ratio of the spatial peak to spatial average intensity.

Bidirectional. Indicating doppler instruments capable of distinguishing between positive and negative doppler shifts (forward and reverse flow).

Bistable. Having two possible states (e.g., on or off; white or black).

Bistable display. Display in which all recorded spots have the same brightness.

Bit. Binary digit.

Cathode ray tube. A display device that produces an image by scanning an electron beam over a phosphor-coated screen.

Cavitation. Production and behavior of bubbles in sound.

Color-flow. The presentation of two-dimensional, real-time doppler shift information superimposed on a real-time, gray-scale anatomic cross-sectional image. Flow directions toward and away from the transducer, i.e., positive and negative doppler shifts, are presented as different colors on the display.

Compensation. Equalizing received reflection amplitude differences caused by reflector depth.

Compressibility. Ability of a material to be reduced to a smaller volume under external pressure.

Compression. Decreasing differences between small and large amplitudes.

Continuous mode. Continuous-wave mode.

Continuous wave. A wave in which cycles repeat indefinitely; not pulsed.

Continuous-wave mode. Mode of operation in which continuous-wave sound is used.

Contrast resolution. Ability of a gray-scale display to distinguish between echoes of slightly different amplitude or intensity.

cos. Abbreviation for cosine.

Cosine. The cosine of angle A in Figure C.1 (Appendix C) is the length of side b divided by the length of side c.

Coupling medium. Oil or gel used to provide a good sound path between the transducer and the skin.

cw. Abbreviation for continuous wave.

Cycle. Complete variation of an acoustic variable.

Damping. Material placed behind the rear face of a transducer element to reduce pulse duration; also, the process of pulse duration reduction.

dB. Abbreviation for decibel.

Dead zone. Region close to the transducer in which imaging cannot be performed.

Decibel. Unit of power or intensity ratio; the number of decibels is 10 times the logarithm (to the base 10) of the power or intensity ratio.

Demodulation. Converting voltage pulses from one form to another.

Density. Mass divided by volume.

Digital. Related to a procedure or system in which data are represented by discrete units (numerical digits).

Disc. Thin flat circular object.

Displacement. Distance that an object has moved.

Doppler angle. The angle between the sound beam and the flow direction.

Doppler effect. Frequency change of reflected sound wave as a result of reflector motion relative to transducer.

Doppler shift. Reflected frequency minus incident frequency.

Duty factor. Fraction of time that pulsed ultrasound is actually on.

Dynamic focusing. Continuously variable received focus that follows the changing position of the transmitted pulse.

Dynamic imaging. Rapid-frame-sequence imaging.

Dynamic range. Ratio (in decibels) of largest power to smallest power that a system can handle or of the largest to the smallest intensity of a group of echoes.

Echo. Reflection.

Effective reflecting area. The area of a reflector from which sound is received by a transducer.

Electric current. The rate of flow of electrons in an electric conductor.

Electric pulse. A brief excursion of electric voltage from its normal value.

Electric resistance. The characteristic of electric components that limits the electric current for a given voltage.

Electric resistor. A device that limits the electric current for a given voltage.

Electric voltage. Electric potential or potential difference expressed in volts.

Electricity. A form of energy associated with the displacement or flow of electrons.

Energy. Capability of doing work.

Enhancement. Increase in reflection amplitude from reflectors that lie behind a weakly attenuating structure.

Far zone. The region of a sound beam in which the beam diameter increases as the distance from the transducer increases.

Focal length. Distance from focused transducer to center of focal region or to the location of the spatial peak intensity.

Focal region. Region of minimum beam diameter and area.

Focus. To concentrate the sound beam into a smaller beam area than would exist otherwise.

Force. That which changes the state of rest or motion of an object.

Fourier transform. A mathematical technique for obtaining a doppler frequency spectrum.

Fractional bandwidth. Bandwidth divided by operating frequency.

Frame. Display image produced by one complete scan of the sound beam.

Frame rate. Number of frames displayed per unit time.

Frequency. Number of cycles per unit time.

Frequency spectrum. The range of frequencies present. In a doppler instrument, the range of doppler shift frequencies present in the returning echoes.

Gain. Ratio of output to input electrical power.

Generator gate. The electronic portion of a pulsed doppler system that converts the continuous voltage of the voltage generator to a pulsed voltage.

Grating lobes. Additional minor beams of sound traveling out in directions different from the primary beam. These result from the multielement structure of transducer arrays.

Gray scale. Continuous range of brightnesses between white and black.

Gray-scale display. Display in which several values of spot brightness may be displayed.

Half-intensity depth. Depth in tissue at which intensity is reduced to one half what it was at the surface.

Heat. Energy resulting from thermal molecular motion.

Hertz. Unit of frequency, one cycle per second; unit of pulse repetition frequency, one pulse per second.

Hydrophone. A small transducer element mounted on the end of a narrow tube.

Hz. Abbreviation for hertz.

Impedance. Density multiplied by sound propagation speed.

Incidence angle. Angle between incident sound direction and line perpendicular to boundary of the medium.

Intensity. Power divided by area.

Intensity reflection coefficient. Reflected intensity divided by incident intensity.

Intensity transmission coefficient. Transmitted intensity divided by incident intensity.

Internal focus. A focus produced by a curved transducer element.

kHz. Abbreviation for kilohertz.

Kilohertz. One thousand hertz.

Lateral. Perpendicular to the direction of sound travel.

Lateral resolution. Minimum reflector separation perpendicular to the sound path required for separate reflections to be produced.

Linear array. Array made up of rectangular elements in a line.

Linear phased array. Linear array operated by applying voltage pulses to all elements, but with small time differences.

Linear switched array. Linear array operated by applying voltage pulses to groups of elements sequentially.

log. Abbreviation for logarithm.

Logarithm. The logarithm (to the base of 10) of a number is equal to the number of tens that must be multiplied together to result in that number.

Longitudinal wave. Wave in which the particle motion is parallel to the direction of wave travel (compressional wave).

M mode. Mode of operation in which the display presents a spot brightening for each pulse delivered from the receiver, producing a two-dimensional recording of reflector position (motion) versus time.

Mass. Measure of an object's resistance to acceleration.

Matching layer. Material placed in front of the front face of a transducer element to reduce the reflection at the transducer surface.

Medium. Material through which a wave travels.

Megahertz. One million hertz.

MHz. Abbreviation for megahertz.

Multipath. Paths to and from a reflector are not the same.

Multiple reflection. Several reflections produced by a pulse encountering a pair of reflectors.

Near zone. The region of a sound beam in which the beam diameter decreases as the distance from the transducer increases.

Oblique incidence. Sound direction is not perpendicular to media boundary.

Operating frequency. Preferred frequency of operation of a transducer.

Particle. Small portion of a medium.

Particle motion. Displacement, speed, velocity, and acceleration of a particle.

Period. Time per cycle.

Perpendicular. Geometrically related by 90 degrees.

Perpendicular incidence. Sound direction is perpendicular to media boundary.

Phantom. Tissue-equivalent materials that have some characteristics representative of tissues (e.g., scattering or attenuation properties).

Piezoelectricity. Conversion of pressure to electric voltage.

Pixel. Picture element; the unit into which imaging information is divided for storage and display in a digital instrument.

Power. Rate at which work is done; rate at which energy is transferred.

Pressure. Force divided by area.

Probe. Transducer assembly.

Propagation. Progression or travel.

Propagation speed. Speed with which a wave moves through a medium.

Pulse. A brief excursion of a quantity from its normal value; a few cycles.

Pulse duration. Time from beginning to end of a pulse.

Pulse-echo diagnostic ultrasound. Ultrasound imaging in which pulses are reflected and used to produce a display.

Pulse repetition frequency. Number of pulses per unit time. Sometimes called pulse repetition rate.

Pulse repetition period. Time from the beginning of one pulse to the beginning of the next.

Pulsed mode. Mode of operation in which pulsed ultrasound is used.

Pulsed ultrasound. Ultrasound produced in pulse form by applying electric pulses to the transducer.

Q factor. Quality factor.

Quality factor. Operating frequency divided by bandwidth.

Range equation. Relationship between round-trip pulse travel time and distance to a reflector.

Rayl. Unit of impedance.

Real-time. Imaging with a rapid-frame-sequence display.

Real-time display. A display that continuously images moving structures or changing scan plane.

Receiver gate. A device that allows only echoes from a selected depth (arrival time) to pass.

Reflection. Portion of sound returned from a boundary of a medium.

Reflection angle. Angle between reflected sound direction and a line perpendicular to the boundary of a medium.

Reflector. Medium boundary that produces a reflection; reflecting surface.

Refraction. Change of sound direction on passing from one medium to another.

Rejection. Eliminating smaller-amplitude voltage pulses.

Resonance frequency. Operating frequency.

Reverberation. Multiple reflections.

Scan converter. A device that stores imaging information in one scanning format and reads it out for display in another.

Scan line. A line produced on a display by moving a spot (produced by an electron beam) across the display face at constant speed.

Scanning. Sweeping a sound beam to produce an image.

Scatterer. An object that scatters sound because of its small size or its surface roughness.

Scattering. Diffusion or redirection of sound in several directions on encountering a particle suspension or a rough surface.

Sensitivity. Ability of an imaging system to detect weak reflections.

Shadowing. Reduction in reflection amplitude from reflectors that lie behind a strongly reflecting or attenuating structure.

Side lobes. Minor beams of sound traveling out in directions different from the primary beam.

sin. Abbreviation for sine.

Sine. The sine of angle A in Figure C.1 (Appendix C) is the length of side a divided by the length of side c.

Sound. Traveling wave of acoustic variables.

Sound beam. The region of a medium that contains virtually all the sound produced by a transducer.

Spatial pulse length. Length of space over which a pulse occurs.

Speckle. The granular appearance of images caused by the interference of echoes from the distribution of scatterers in tissue.

Spectral broadening. The widening of the doppler shift spectrum, i.e., the increase of the range of doppler shift frequencies present, owing to a broader range of flow speeds encountered by the sound beam. This occurs for normal flow in smaller vessels and for turbulent flow in any vessel.

Specular reflection. Reflection from a smooth boundary.

Speed. Displacement divided by time over which displacement occurs.

Stiffness. Property of a medium; applied pressure divided by fractional volume change produced by the pressure.

Strength. Nonspecific term referring to amplitude or intensity.

Temperature. Condition of a body that determines transfer of heat to or from other bodies.

Test object. A device designed to measure some characteristic of an imaging system without having tissue-like properties.

TGC. Compensation; time gain compensation.

Transducer. Device that converts energy from one form to another.

Transducer array. Transducer assembly containing more than one transducer element.

Transducer assembly. Transducer element with damping and matching materials assembled in a case.

Transducer element. Piece of piezoelectric material in a transducer assembly.

Transmission angle. Angle between transmitted sound direction and a line perpendicular to the boundary of a medium.

Ultrasound. Sound of frequency greater than 20 kHz.

Ultrasound transducer. Device that converts electric energy to ultrasound energy and vice versa.

Variable focusing. Transmit focus with various focal lengths.

Velocity. Speed with direction of motion specified.

Voltage pulse. Brief excursion of voltage from its normal value.

Wave. Traveling variation of wave variables.

Wave variables. Things that are functions of space and time in a wave.

Wavelength. Length of space over which a cycle occurs.

Work. Force multiplied by displacement.

Answers to Exercises in the Text

Chapter 1

1.1 pulses, ultrasound, echoes, image
1.2 pulse, echo
1.3 strength
1.4 parallel
1.5 origin (starting point)
1.6 rectangular
1.7 pie
1.8 doppler, flow
1.9 frequency
1.10 pulse, echo, location, strength, location, brightness
1.11 65 μs (13 μs/cm x 5 cm)

Chapter 2

2.2.1 wave variables
2.2.2 acoustic variables

270

2.2.3 20,000
2.2.4 pressure, density, temperature, particle motion
2.2.5 c, d, e
2.2.6 a, e
2.2.7 cycles
2.2.8 hertz, Hz
2.2.9 time
2.2.10 frequency
2.2.11 space
2.2.12 wave
2.2.13 propagation speed, frequency
2.2.14 density, stiffness
2.2.15 e
2.2.16 1540, 1.54
2.2.17 e
2.2.18 a, c, b
2.2.19 1.54
2.2.20 decreases
2.2.21 10
2.2.22 higher
2.2.23 d
2.2.24 b
2.2.25 higher
2.2.26 mechanical longitudinal
2.2.27 doubled
2.2.28 1
2.2.29 unchanged
2.2.30 energy, information
2.2.31 e
2.2.32 false
2.2.33 true
2.2.34 1,540,000 (propagation speed is 1540 m/s)
2.2.35 true
2.2.36 true
2.2.37 density, propagation speed
2.2.38 a. 0.1 μs, 10 MHz
       b. 0.25 ms, 4 MHz
2.2.39 1.54
2.2.40 0.385

2.3.1 continuous wave
2.3.2 pulses
2.3.3 pulses

2.3.4 pulses
2.3.5 period
2.3.6 over
2.3.7 time
2.3.8 length, space
2.3.9 duty factor
2.3.10 period
2.3.11 wavelength
2.3.12 1 (100 per cent)
2.3.13 6
2.3.14 2
2.3.15 1.3 (period is 0.33 μs, soft tissue is irrelevant)
2.3.16 1
2.3.17 0.0013
2.3.18 d
2.3.19 c
2.3.20 b
2.3.21 less than

2.4.1 variation
2.4.2 power, area
2.4.3 W/cm^2
2.4.4 amplitude
2.4.5 doubled
2.4.6 halved
2.4.7 unchanged
2.4.8 quadrupled
2.4.9 5
2.4.10 peak, average
2.4.11 average, pulse
2.4.12 b
2.4.13 a. 3; b. 1; c. 3
2.4.14 2
2.4.15 3, 4
2.4.16 amplitude, intensity
2.4.17 absorption, reflection, scattering
2.4.18 length
2.4.19 dB, dB/cm
2.4.20 0.5
2.4.21 1.5 dB/cm
2.4.22 increases
2.4.23 doubled, doubled, quadrupled
2.4.24 unchanged

2.4.25 sound, heat
2.4.26 no (absorption is one part of attenuation)
2.4.27 higher
2.4.28 50, 1.5, 50, 1
2.4.29 0.6
2.4.30 2.5
2.4.31 attenuation coefficient, frequency
2.4.32 decreases
2.4.33 0.32 (intensity ratio is 0.16), 1.5
2.4.34 0.00000002
2.4.35 c

2.5.1 impedances
2.5.2 impedances, intensity
2.5.3 impedances
2.5.4 0.0008, 1.9992
2.5.5 0.0002, 1.9998
2.5.6 0.0008, 1.9992
2.5.7 0.01, 1 (incident intensity not needed)
2.5.8 0.99, 99
2.5.9 20 (intensity ratio 0.01, use Table C.2 in Appendix C)
2.5.10 0.01
2.5.11 0 (impedances are equal)
2.5.12 5, 0
2.5.13 true
2.5.14 false, in general (true only if propagation speeds are also equal)
2.5.15 false, in general (true only if densities are also equal)
2.5.16 false
2.5.17 0.9990
2.5.18 air, reflection
2.5.19 0.01
2.5.20 0.43
2.5.21 d
2.5.22 direction
2.5.23 larger than, equal to
2.5.24 smaller than, equal to
2.5.25 equal to, equal to
2.5.26 30, 21
2.5.27 30, 30
2.5.28 30, 39
2.5.29 0.04 (incidence angle and intensity are not needed; the propagation speeds are equal, so that the calculation is the same as with perpendicular incidence)

2.5.30 0.2 (no refraction; calculate as with perpendicular incidence)
2.5.31 perpendicular incidence, media propagation speeds are equal
2.5.32 media propagation speeds are equal (no refraction)
2.5.33 density, propagation speed
2.5.34 32
2.5.35 1.7
2.5.36 scattering
2.5.37 true
2.5.38 false
2.5.39 a
2.5.40 true
2.5.41 c
2.5.42 pulses, echoes, display
2.5.43 propagation speed, time
2.5.44 4
2.5.45 7
2.5.46 7.7
2.5.47 1
2.5.48 3
2.5.49 10

2.6.1 a
2.6.2 e
2.6.3 a. 4; b.1; c. 3; d. 5; e. 2
2.6.4 a. 2; b. 3; c. 4; d. 1
2.6.5 a. 3; b. 4, c. 1; d. 2; e. 5; f. 7; g. 6
2.6.6 a. 3; b. 4; c. 1; d. 2; e. 1; f. 3; g. 1; h. 5; i. 8; j. 7; k. 6; l. 9; m. 4
2.6.7 a. 1; b. 2, 3; c. 3, d. 1; e. 2
2.6.8 a. 1.54; b. 0.77; c. 3.1; d. 0.5; e. 2; f. 1; g. 0.002; h. 2; i. 1; j. 3.0; k. 6; l. 0.25; m. 0.25; n. 1; o. 125; p. 500; q. 1,630,000
2.6.9 c
2.6.10 a
2.6.11 increased
2.6.12 100 μs, 50 μs, 0.5, 10 kHz, 17 μs, 60 kHz
2.6.13 propagation speeds, equal
2.6.14 d
2.6.15 e
2.6.16 d
2.6.17 0.04
2.6.18 impedances
2.6.19 densities or impedances, propagation speeds
2.6.20 18
2.6.21 23

2.6.22 false
2.6.23 80

Chapter 3

3.2.1 energy
3.2.2 electrical, ultrasound
3.2.3 piezoelectricity
3.2.4 discs
3.2.5 thickness
3.2.6 element, assembly
3.2.7 element, assembly
3.2.8 continuous-wave
3.2.9 pulses
3.2.10 decreases
3.2.11 cycle, axial resolution, bandwidth, quality factor
3.2.12 efficiency, sensitivity
3.2.13 two, three
3.2.14 0.2
3.2.15 15
3.2.16 reflection
3.2.17 air
3.2.18 e
3.2.19 false
3.2.20 frequencies
3.2.21 c
3.2.22 a. 3; b. 0.33; c. 2.5; d. 3.5; e. 3

3.3.1 4
3.3.2 near, far
3.3.3 near-zone
3.3.4 frequency or wavelength, diameter, distance
3.3.5 transducer diameter, wavelength
3.3.6 transducer diameter, frequency
3.3.7 one half
3.3.8 two
3.3.9 decreases
3.3.10 increases
3.3.11 30
3.3.12 4.5, 3, 6, 12
3.3.13 60
3.3.14 3, 6, 9

3.3.15 longer, smaller
3.3.16 120
3.3.17 9, 6, 9, 12
3.3.18 longer, smaller
3.3.19 quadruples
3.3.20 doubles
3.3.21 doubled
3.3.22 e
3.3.23 false
3.3.24 focal length

3.4.1 element
3.4.2 linear, annular
3.4.3 switched, phased
3.4.4 a. 1; b. 2, 3; c. 2, 3; d. 3, 1, 2; e. 1, 2, 3
3.4.5 one
3.4.6 two
3.4.7 oscillating mirror
3.4.8 a. 1; b. 2; c. 2
3.4.9 b
3.4.10 a
3.4.11 c

3.5.1 sound travel, reflections
3.5.2 spatial pulse length
3.5.3 true
3.5.4 1.5
3.5.5 1
3.5.6 2.3, 0.2
3.5.7 halved
3.5.8 doubled
3.5.9 false
3.5.10 false
3.5.11 1
3.5.12 10 (less than 10 MHz in many applications)
3.5.13 wavelength, spatial pulse length
3.5.14 attenuation
3.5.15 separation, reflections
3.5.16 beam diameter or width
3.5.17 c, d, f
3.5.18 true

3.5.19 true
3.5.20 false (only true near the transducer)
3.5.21 b, c, e, f

3.6.1 a. 4; b. 3; c. 2; d. 1
3.6.2 a, d
3.6.3 a. 5; b. 0.3; c. 141; d. 6.5; e. 13
3.6.4 c
3.6.5 one half, near-zone
3.6.6 focal
3.6.7 6.5 (frequency not needed)
3.6.8 0.7 (diameter not needed)
3.6.9 true
3.6.10 false
3.6.11 focal
3.6.12 true
3.6.13 false
3.6.14 a. 1, 2, 3; b. 2; c. 2; d. 1
3.6.15 a
3.6.16 e
3.6.17 a
3.6.18 b, c, d
3.6.19 true
3.6.20 resolution, imaging depth
3.6.21 1, 10
3.6.22 1, 1.5
3.6.23 2 (or possibly 1) mm
3.6.24 4 cm
3.6.25 2 or 3 mm

Chapter 4

4.1.1 pulser, transducer, receiver, memory, display
4.1.2 a. 4; b. 1; c. 2; d. 5; e. 3
4.1.3 a. 2; b. 2; c. 2, 3; d. 3; e. 1; f. 1; g. 2; h. 1, 2; i. 2, 3; j. 2, 3; k. 1, 2; l. 1, 2; m. 2, 3; n. 2, 3; o. 2, 3; p. 2, 3

4.2.1 pulse
4.2.2 amplitude, intensity
4.2.3 a. 3; b. 5; c. 1; d. 2; e. 4

4.3.1 amplification, compensation, compression, demodulation, rejection

4.3.2 a. 2; b. 5; c. 3; d. 1; e. 4

4.3.3 10, 100, 20

4.3.4 1

4.3.5 10

4.3.6 b, e

4.3.7 depth, distance

4.3.8 times

4.3.9 dynamic, display

4.3.10 2.0

4.3.11 pulses

4.3.12 false

4.3.13 a

4.4.1 a. 5; b. 3; c. 2; d. 1; e. 4

4.4.2 a

4.4.3 c

4.4.4 a. 5; b. 3; c. 2; d. 6; e. 1; f. 4

4.4.5 e

4.4.6 a. 4; b. 5; c. 6; d. 7; e. 8

4.4.7 d

4.4.8 d

4.4.9 e

4.4.10 a

4.5.1 A, B, M, B

4.5.2 a. 2, 7; b. 3, 7; c. 3, 4, 7; d. 1, 3, 5, 6

4.5.3 cathode ray

4.5.4 deflection

4.5.5 time, distance or depth

4.5.6 true

4.5.7 M

4.5.8 time, propagation speed

4.5.9 scanning

4.5.10 gray-scale

4.5.11 scan converter

4.5.12 c

4.5.13 d

4.5.14 33

4.5.15 63

4.5.16 a. 1; b. 2; c. 2; d. 2; e.1; f. 2

4.5.17 40

4.5.18 1200
4.5.19 4, 4
4.5.20 0.4, 0.4

4.6.1 a
4.6.2 b
4.6.3 d
4.6.4 c
4.6.5 d
4.6.6 b, f, e, d, c, a
4.6.7 b
4.6.8 b
4.6.9 d
4.6.10 2, 60
4.6.11 b
4.6.12 reflections or echoes
4.6.13 reflection or pulse-echo
4.6.14 pulse-echo
4.6.15 strength, direction, time
4.6.16 a
4.6.17 display, voltages or pulses
4.6.18 receiver
4.6.19 pulser
4.6.20 receiver
4.6.21 a
4.6.22 f
4.6.23 b
4.6.24 e
4.6.25 c
4.6.26 d
4.6.27 c
4.6.28 b
4.6.29 a
4.6.30 false
4.6.31 A, M
4.6.32 B
4.6.33 mechanical, electronic
4.6.34 frame
4.6.35 pulsed
4.6.36 lines, frame
4.6.37 false (latter portion)
4.6.38 increase
4.6.39 improved, decreases, increased

4.6.40 512 x 512 = 262,144
4.6.41 b, a, c
4.6.42 a and c
4.6.43 1000/20 = 50 lines per frame (one scan line for each pulse)

Chapter 5

5.6.1 5.1
5.6.2 77
5.6.3 c
5.6.4 false
5.6.5 e
5.6.6 a
5.6.7 false. This is the display of the interference pattern of scattered sound from the distribution of scatterers in the tissue.
5.6.8 section thickness
5.6.9 c, d, e, f
5.6.10 true
5.6.11 5.8
5.6.12 a. 1; b. 2, 3; c. 3; d. 3; e. 2, 3; f. 4, 5; g. 4, 5; h. 4; i. 2,6
5.6.13 separation
5.6.14 weaker
5.6.15 b
5.6.16 d
5.6.17 true
5.6.18 b
5.6.19 192
5.6.20 3.8
5.6.21 no (200 x 25 x 20 = 100,000; greater than 77,000)
5.6.22 refraction (double image)

Chapter 6

6.2.1 frequency or wavelength motion
6.2.2 higher
6.2.3 lower
6.2.4 equal to
6.2.5 motion
6.2.6 0.02, 1.02
6.2.7 0.026
6.2.8 -0.026

6.2.9 reflected, incident
6.2.10 cosine
6.2.11 0.01, 1.01 (the doppler shift is cut in half)
6.2.12 0, 1.00 (no doppler shift at 90 degrees)
6.2.13 110

6.3.1 false
6.3.2 direction, bidirectional
6.3.3 false
6.3.4 voltage generator, source transducer, receiving transducer, receiver, loudspeaker
6.3.5 amplitude, frequency
6.3.6 frequency, time
6.3.7 gray, color
6.3.8 flow velocities
6.3.9 true

6.4.1 gates, transducers
6.4.2 continuous, pulsed
6.4.3 depths, arrival time
6.4.4 false
6.4.5 profile
6.4.6 true
6.4.7 a
6.4.8 gates

6.5.1 flow, anatomy
6.5.2 d
6.5.3 red, blue, blue, red
6.5.4 autocorrelation, mean
6.5.5 b

6.6.1 doppler shift
6.6.2 false
6.6.3 one, two
6.6.4 frequencies
6.6.5 false
6.6.6 motion
6.6.7 gate
6.6.8 display
6.6.9 gate, voltage generator
6.6.10 depth
6.6.11 true

6.6.12 false
6.6.13 true
6.6.14 2.6
6.6.15 true
6.6.16 continuous wave
6.6.17 b

Chapter 7

7.2.1 rods, water, alcohol
7.2.2 a. 1; b. 2; c. 3; d. 6; e. 4; f. 3; g. 7; h. 7
7.2.3 a. 5; b. 5; c. 4; d. 3; e. 2; f. 1; g. 1; h. 1
7.2.4 true
7.2.5 true
7.2.6 1
7.2.7 distance
7.2.8 distances or depths
7.2.9 tissues
7.2.10 false
7.2.11 d
7.2.12 false
7.2.13 b
7.2.14 d

7.3.1 b, c, d, e
7.3.2 true
7.3.3 transducer
7.3.4 true
7.3.5 b
7.3.6 a. 1, 12 or 1, 9; b. 3, 12; c. 3, 8; d. 4 or 2, 9; e. 1, 7; f. 5, 10; g. 6, 11

7.4.1 a
7.4.2 a
7.4.3 b
7.4.4 e

7.5.1 false
7.5.2 d

7.6.1 a. 2; b. 1, 2; c. 2, 3
7.6.2 a. 2; b. 3; c. 1
7.6.3 false

7.6.4 false
7.6.5 b
7.6.6 no
7.6.7 yes

Chapter 8

8.1 a
8.2 c
8.3 d
8.4 e
8.5 e
8.6 a
8.7 a
8.8 c
8.9 c
8.10 false (only true near the transducer)
8.11 false (only true for normal incidence or oblique incidence when densities and propagation speeds of the media are equal)
8.12 false (see comment for 8.11)
8.13 c
8.14 d
8.15 e (A mode)
8.16 d
8.17 false (6 bits)
8.18 d
8.19 d
8.20 a. 1, 3, 4; b. 2, 5; c. 1, 3, 5
8.21 a
8.22 b
8.23 c
8.24 d (areas are 284 and 3 mm^2)
8.25 c
8.26 d
8.27 e
8.28 c
8.29 d
8.30 d
8.31 c
8.32 c
8.33 b
8.34 Yes

8.35 a
8.36 a
8.37 a
8.38 a
8.39 d (b and c)
8.40 d
8.41 c
8.42 d
8.43 c
8.44 c
8.45 e (d and a or b)
8.46 a. 1, 2; b. 1, 2; c. 2, 3; d. 1, 2, 3
8.47 c
8.48 b
8.49 b
8.50 c
8.51 See p. 285
8.52 See p. 286
8.53 See p. 287
8.54 See p. 288
8.55 a
8.56 e
8.57 a
8.58 b
8.59 b
8.60 d
8.61 b
8.62 a, b, c, d, e
8.63 c
8.64 e
8.65 a
8.66 e
8.67 d
8.68 b
8.69 c
8.70 d
8.71 a
8.72 false
8.73 false
8.74 e
8.75 b
8.76 a. 2; b. 2; c. 1.5 mm; d. 3 mm; e. 10 μs; f. 100 kHz; g. 2 μs; h. 1 μs; i. 1 MHz; j. 0.2; k. 1.5 mm/μs

8.51

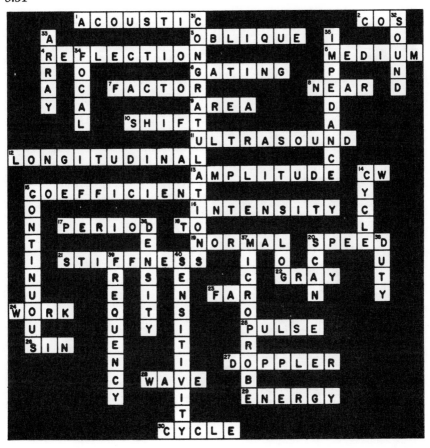

8.52

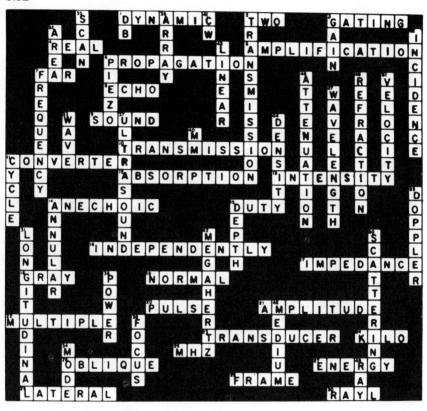

8.53

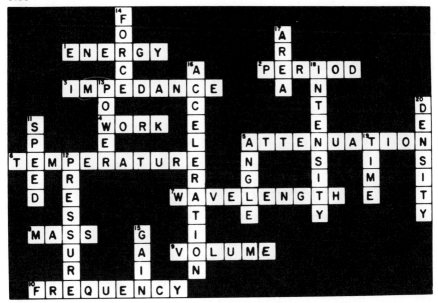

8.77 10, 1, 0.01, 0.01, 0.001

8.78 c, a, b, b

8.79 longer, longer, none; b; a, b, and d

8.80 continuous-wave, 1.5, 1.5, 3

8.81 1, 1, 2, continuous-wave, 1.54

8.82 e

8.83 attenuation, 6, 2, 4

8.84 b

8.85 c

8.86 a

8.87 b

8.88 c

8.89 a, b, g, k, l, o, q, r

8.90 s

8.54

START

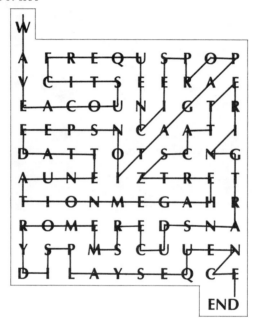

Appendix A
Symbols and Abbreviations

a	attenuation, acceleration
a_c	attenuation coefficient
A	area, current
A_B	beam area
A_P	pressure amplitude
A_V	particle velocity amplitude
ARC	amplitude reflection coefficient
BUR	beam uniformity ratio
BW	bandwidth
c	sound propagation speed
c_m	transducer material propagation speed
d	distance to reflector displacement
d_m	maximum unambiguous imaging depth
D	half-intensity depth
D_B	beam diameter
D_I	imaging depth
D_T	transducer diameter
DF	duty factor
E	energy

f	frequency
f_D	doppler shift
f_i	incident frequency
f_o	operating frequency
f_r	reflected frequency
F	force
FBW	fractional bandwidth
FR	frame rate
I	intensity, current
I_i	incident intensity
I_r	reflected intensity
I_t	transmitted intensity
I_{SA}	spatial average intensity
I_{SP}	spatial peak intensity
I_{TA}	temporal average intensity
I_{PA}	pulse average intensity
IRC	intensity reflection coefficient
ITC	intensity transmission coefficient
l	path length
LD	line density
LPF	lines per frame
m	mass
M	stiffness
n	number of cycles in a pulse
NZL	near-zone length
p	pressure
P	power
PD	pulse duration
PRF	pulse repetition frequency
PRP	pulse repetition period
Q	quality factor
R	resistance
R_A	axial resolution
R_L	lateral resolution
s	speed
S_r	reflector speed
SA	sector angle
SPL	spatial pulse length
t	time, pulse round-trip time
T	period
v	velocity
V	volume, voltage
w	transducer thickness

W	work
W_d	display width
z	impedance
Δv	velocity change
ΔV_F	fractional volume change
λ	wavelength
ρ	density
θ	doppler angle
θ_i	incidence angle
θ_r	reflection angle
θ_t	transmission angle

Appendix B
Equations

For convenient reference, the 40 equations presented throughout this book (excluding the appendices) are compiled here. One asterisk over the equals symbol indicates that the equation is specifically for soft tissues. Two asterisks over the equals symbol indicate that the equation is specifically for perpendicular incidence. The ten most fundamental and important equations are indicated with arrows ($\leftarrow$).

Chapter 2

$$\text{period (}\mu\text{s)} = \frac{1}{\text{frequency (MHz)}} \qquad\qquad T = \frac{1}{f}$$

$$\text{wavelength (mm)} = \frac{\text{propagation speed (mm/}\mu\text{s)}}{\text{frequency (MHz)}} \qquad\qquad \lambda = \frac{c}{f} \qquad \leftarrow 1$$

$$\text{wavelength (mm)} \overset{*}{=} \frac{1.54}{\text{frequency (MHz)}} \qquad\qquad \lambda \overset{*}{=} \frac{1.54}{f}$$

impedance = density x propagation speed $z = \rho c$ ← 2
  (rayl)   (kg/m³)   (m/s)

$$\text{pulse repetition period (ms)} = \frac{1}{\text{pulse repetition frequency (kHz)}} \qquad PRP = \frac{1}{PRF}$$

$$\text{pulse duration (µs)} = \frac{\text{number of cycles}}{\text{in the pulse}} \times \text{period (µs)} \qquad PD = nT$$

$$\text{pulse duration (µs)} = \frac{\text{number of cycles in the pulse}}{\text{frequency (MHz)}} \qquad PD = \frac{n}{f}$$

$$\text{duty factor} = \frac{\text{pulse duration (µs)}}{\text{pulse repetition period (ms) x 1000}} \qquad DF = \frac{PD}{PRP \times 1000} \quad ← 3$$

$$\text{duty factor} = \frac{\text{pulse duration (µs)} \times \text{pulse repetition frequency (kHz)}}{1000} \qquad DF = \frac{PD \times PRF}{1000}$$

$$\text{spatial pulse length (mm)} = \frac{\text{number of cycles in the pulse}}{\text{x wavelength (mm)}} \qquad SPL = n\lambda$$

$$\text{spatial pulse length (mm)} = \frac{\text{number of cycles in the pulse} \times \text{propagation speed (mm/µs)}}{\text{frequency (MHz)}} \qquad SPL = \frac{nc}{f}$$

$$\text{spatial pulse length (mm)} \overset{*}{=} \frac{\text{number of cycles in the pulse} \times 1.54}{\text{frequency (MHz)}} \qquad SPL \overset{*}{=} \frac{n \times 1.54}{f}$$

$$\text{intensity (W/cm}^2) = \frac{\text{power (W)}}{\text{area (cm}^2)} \qquad I = \frac{P}{A} \quad ← 4$$

$$\text{spatial average intensity (W/cm}^2) = \frac{\text{spatial peak intensity (W/cm}^2)}{\text{beam uniformity ratio}} \qquad I_{SA} = \frac{I_{SP}}{BUR}$$

$$\text{temporal average intensity (W/cm}^2) = \text{duty factor} \times \text{pulse average intensity (W/cm}^2) \qquad I_{TA} = DF \times I_{PA}$$

$$\text{attenuation (dB)} = \frac{\text{attenuation coefficient (dB/cm)}}{\times \text{ path length (cm)}} \qquad a = a_c l$$

$$\text{attenuation (dB)} \overset{*}{=} \tfrac{1}{2} \times \text{ frequency (MHz)} \times \text{ path length (cm)} \quad a \overset{*}{=} \tfrac{1}{2}fl \qquad \leftarrow 5$$

$$\text{half-intensity depth (cm)} = \frac{3}{\text{attenuation coefficient (dB/cm)}} \qquad D = \frac{3}{a_c}$$

$$\text{half-intensity depth (cm)} \overset{*}{=} \frac{6}{\text{frequency (MHz)}} \qquad D \overset{*}{=} \frac{6}{f}$$

$$\begin{matrix}\text{intensity reflection} \\ \text{coefficient}\end{matrix} = \frac{\text{reflected intensity (W/cm}^2)}{\text{incident intensity (W/cm}^2)} \qquad IRC = \frac{I_r}{I_i}$$

$$\overset{**}{=} \left[\frac{\text{medium two impedance} - \text{medium one impedance}}{\text{medium two impedance} + \text{medium one impedance}}\right]^2 \quad \overset{**}{=} \left[\frac{z_2 - z_1}{z_2 + z_1}\right]^2 \leftarrow 6$$

$$\begin{matrix}\text{intensity transmission} \\ \text{coefficient}\end{matrix} = \frac{\text{transmitted intensity (W/cm}^2)}{\text{incident intensity (W/cm}^2)} \qquad ITC = \frac{I_t}{I_i}$$

$$\overset{**}{=} 1 - \text{intensity reflection coefficient} \qquad \overset{**}{=} 1 - IRC$$

$$\text{reflection angle (°)} = \text{incidence angle (°)} \qquad \theta_r = \theta_i$$

$$\begin{matrix}\text{transmission} \\ \text{angle (°)}\end{matrix} = \begin{matrix}\text{incidence} \\ \text{angle (°)}\end{matrix} \times \left[\frac{\begin{matrix}\text{medium two} \\ \text{propagation speed (mm/µs)}\end{matrix}}{\begin{matrix}\text{medium one} \\ \text{propagation speed (mm/µs)}\end{matrix}}\right] \qquad \theta_t = \theta_i\left[\frac{c_2}{c_1}\right]$$

$$\begin{matrix}\text{distance to} \\ \text{reflector (mm)}\end{matrix} = \begin{matrix}\tfrac{1}{2}[\text{propagation speed (mm/µs)} \\ \times \text{ pulse round-trip time (µs)}]\end{matrix} \qquad d = \tfrac{1}{2}ct$$

$$\begin{matrix}\text{distance to} \\ \text{reflector (mm)}\end{matrix} \overset{*}{=} 0.77 \times \text{ pulse round-trip time (µs)} \qquad d \overset{*}{=} 0.77t \qquad \leftarrow 7$$

Chapter 3

$$\text{operating frequency (MHz)} = \frac{\text{propagation speed (mm/µs)}}{2 \times \text{ thickness (mm)}} \qquad f_o = \frac{c_m}{2w}$$

quality factor $= \dfrac{\text{operating frequency (MHz)}}{\text{bandwidth (MHz)}}$ $Q = \dfrac{f_o}{BW}$

near-zone length (mm) $= \dfrac{[\text{transducer diameter (mm)}]^2}{4 \times \text{wavelength (mm)}}$ $NZL = \dfrac{D_T^2}{4\lambda}$

$\dfrac{\text{near-zone}}{\text{length (mm)}} \overset{*}{=} \dfrac{[\text{transducer diameter (mm)}]^2 \times \text{frequency (MHz)}}{6}$ $NZL \overset{*}{=} \dfrac{D_T^2 f}{6}$ $\leftarrow 8$

beam area (cm²) $= 0.8 \times [\text{beam diameter (cm)}^2]$ $A_B = 0.8\,D_B^2$

axial resolution $= \dfrac{\text{spatial pulse length (mm)}}{2}$ $R_A = \dfrac{SPL}{2}$ $\leftarrow 9$

axial resolution $\overset{*}{=} \dfrac{0.77 \times \text{number of cycles in the pulse}}{\text{frequency (MHz)}}$ $R_A \overset{*}{=} \dfrac{0.77n}{f}$

lateral resolution (mm) = beam diameter (mm) $R_L = D_B$ $\leftarrow 10$

Chapter 4

$\dfrac{\text{pulse repetition}}{\text{frequency (Hz)}} =$ lines per frame $\times$ frame rate $PRF = LPF \times FR$

line density (lines/cm) $= \dfrac{\text{lines per frame}}{\text{display width (cm)}}$ $LD = \dfrac{LPF}{W_d}$

line density (lines/degree) $= \dfrac{\text{lines per frame}}{\text{sector angle (degrees)}}$ $LD = \dfrac{LPF}{SA}$

Chapter 5

maximum depth (cm) $= \dfrac{77}{\text{pulse repetition frequency (kHz)}}$ $d_m = \dfrac{77}{PRF}$

$$\frac{\text{maximum}}{\text{depth (cm)}} \times \frac{\text{lines}}{\text{per frame}} \times \frac{\text{frame}}{\text{rate}} = 77{,}000 \qquad\qquad \frac{d_m \times \text{LPF}}{\times \text{FR} = 77{,}000}$$

Chapter 6

doppler shift (MHz) = reflected frequency (MHz) - incident frequency (MHz)

$$= \pm\ \frac{2\ \times\ \text{reflector speed (m/s)}\ \times\ \text{incident frequency (MHz)}}{\text{propagation speed (m/s)}}$$

$$f_D = f_r - f_i = \pm\ \frac{2\ \times\ S_r \times\ f_i}{c}$$

Appendix C
Mathematics

C.1
Algebra

Only the basic mathematical concepts that are applicable to the material in this book will be considered in this appendix.

Transposition of quantities in algebraic equations is accomplished by performing identical mathematical operations on both sides.

Example C.1.1

For the equation

$$x + y = z$$

transpose to get x alone (solve for x). To do this, subtract y from both sides:

$$x + y - y = z - y$$

Since y − y = 0, the left-hand side of the equation is

$$x + y - y = x + 0 = x$$

so that

$$x = z - y$$

Example C.1.2

For the equation

$$x - y = z$$

solve for x. Add y to both sides:

$$x - y + y = z + y$$
$$x + 0 = z + y$$
$$x = z + y$$

Example C.1.3

For the equation

$$xy = z$$

solve for x. Divide both sides by y:

$$\frac{xy}{y} = \frac{z}{y}$$

Since $\dfrac{y}{y} = 1$

$$\frac{xy}{y} = x(1) = x$$

and

$$x = \frac{z}{y}$$

Example C.1.4

For the equation

$$\frac{x}{y} = z$$

solve for x. Multiply both sides by y:

$$\frac{x}{y}y = zy$$

$$x(1) = zy$$

$$x = zy$$

Example C.1.5

Using some numbers, and combining the previous examples, consider the equation

$$\frac{5x + 3}{2} - 3 = 1$$

Solve for x. Add 3:

$$\frac{5x + 3}{2} - 3 + 3 = 1 + 3$$

$$\frac{5x + 3}{2} = 4$$

Multiply by 2:

$$\frac{5x + 3}{2} \times 2 = 4 \times 2$$

$$5x + 3 = 8$$

Subtract 3:

$$5x + 3 - 3 = 8 - 3$$

$$5x = 5$$

Divide by 5:

$$x = 1$$

Substitution of the answer into the original equation shows that the equality is satisfied and the answer is correct:

$$\frac{5(1) + 3}{2} - 3 = 1$$

$$\frac{8}{2} - 3 = 1$$

$$4 - 3 = 1$$

$$1 = 1$$

Example C.1.6

For the equation

$$\text{propagation speed} = \text{frequency} \times \text{wavelength}$$

solve for wavelength. Divide by frequency:

$$\frac{\text{propagation speed}}{\text{frequency}} = \frac{\text{frequency} \times \text{wavelength}}{\text{frequency}}$$

$$\frac{\text{propagation speed}}{\text{frequency}} = \text{wavelength}$$

Example C.1.7

If the intensity reflection coefficient is 0.1 and the reflected intensity is 5 mW/cm^2, find the incident intensity, given that

$$\text{intensity reflection coefficient} = \frac{\text{reflected intensity}}{\text{incident intensity}}$$

Multiply by incident intensity:

intensity reflection coefficient $\times$ incident intensity

$$= \frac{\text{reflected intensity}}{\text{incident intensity}} \times \text{incident intensity} = \text{reflected intensity}$$

Divide by intensity reflection coefficient:

$$\frac{\text{intensity reflection coefficient} \times \text{incident intensity}}{\text{intensity reflection coefficient}} = \frac{\text{reflected intensity}}{\text{intensity reflection coefficient}}$$

$$\frac{\text{incident}}{\text{intensity}} = \frac{\text{reflected intensity}}{\text{intensity reflection coefficient}} = \frac{5\,\text{mW/cm}^2}{0.1} = 50\,\text{mW/cm}^2$$

Example C.1.8

If the intensity reflection coefficient is 0.01 and the impedance for medium one is 4.5, find the medium two impedance, given that

intensity reflection coefficient =

$$\left[\frac{\text{medium two impedance} - \text{medium one impedance}}{\text{medium two impedance} + \text{medium one impedance}} \right]^2$$

Take the square root of each side:

$$(\text{intensity reflection coefficient})^{\frac{1}{2}} = \frac{\text{medium two impedance} - \text{medium one impedance}}{\text{medium two impedance} + \text{medium one impedance}}$$

Multiply by the sum of medium two impedance and medium one impedance:

(intensity reflection coefficient)$^{\frac{1}{2}}$ x (medium two impedance + medium one impedance) = medium two impedance - medium one impedance

Add the medium one impedance:

(intensity reflection coefficient)$^{\frac{1}{2}}$ x (medium two impedance + medium one impedance) + medium one impedance = medium two impedance

Subtract (intensity reflection coefficient)$^{\frac{1}{2}}$ x medium two impedance:

[(intensity reflection coefficient)$^{\frac{1}{2}}$ x medium one impedance] + medium one impedance = medium two impedance - [(intensity reflection coefficient)$^{\frac{1}{2}}$ x medium two impedance]

medium one impedance [1 + (intensity reflection coefficient)$^{\frac{1}{2}}$]
= medium two impedance [1 - (intensity reflection coefficient)$^{\frac{1}{2}}$]

Divide by [1 - (intensity reflection coefficient)$^{1/2}$] and interchange sides of the equation:

medium two impedance = medium one impedance

$$\left[\frac{1 + (\text{intensity reflection coefficient})^{1/2}}{1 - (\text{intensity reflection coefficient})^{1/2}} \right]$$

$$= 4.5 \left[\frac{1 + (0.01)^{1/2}}{1 - (0.01)^{1/2}} \right]$$

$$= 4.5 \left[\frac{1 + 0.1}{1 - 0.1} \right] = 4.5 \left[\frac{1.1}{0.9} \right] = 4.5\,(1.22) = 5.5$$

medium two impedance = 5.5

Exercises†

C.1.1 Solve each of the following for x:
   a. x + y + 2 = z
   b. x - y = z - 1
   c. 2xy = z
   d. x/y = 3z
   e. $\dfrac{x + 5}{4}$ - 2 = 4
   f. $\dfrac{3x + 3}{2}$ - 2 = 4

C.1.2 Solve each of the following for the quantity with the asterisk:
   a. propagation speed = frequency* x wavelength
   b. intensity = $\dfrac{\text{power}}{\text{beam area*}}$
   c. period = $\dfrac{1}{\text{frequency*}}$

C.1.3 The age of an ultrasound instrument is equal to three times its age three years from now minus three times its age three years ago. What is its present age?

C.1.4 Let:

$$y + x = \tfrac{1}{2}(7y - 3x)$$

---

† Answers to appendix exercises are given on pages 349 to 351.

Subtract 2x from both sides so that:

$$y - x = \frac{1}{2}(7y - 3x) - 2x$$

Divide both sides by $(y - x)$:

$$\frac{y - x}{y - x} = \frac{7y - 3x}{2(y - x)} - \frac{2x}{y - x}$$

Combine right side into single fraction:

$$\frac{y - x}{y - x} = \frac{7y - 3x - 4x}{2(y - x)} = \frac{7(y - x)}{2(y - x)}$$

Multiply both sides by 2:

$$2 \left[\frac{y - x}{y - x} \right] = 7 \left[\frac{y - x}{y - x} \right]$$

Therefore $2 = 7$. What went wrong?

C.2
Trigonometry

If the sides and angles of a right triangle (one of the angles equals 90 degrees) are labeled as in Figure C.1, the sine of angle A (sin A) and the cosine of angle A (cos A) are defined as follows:

$$\sin A = \frac{\text{length of side a}}{\text{length of side c}}$$

$$\cos A = \frac{\text{length of side b}}{\text{length of side c}}$$

Example C.2.1

If the lengths of the sides a, b, and c are 1, $\sqrt{3}$, and 2, respectively, what are sin A and cos A?

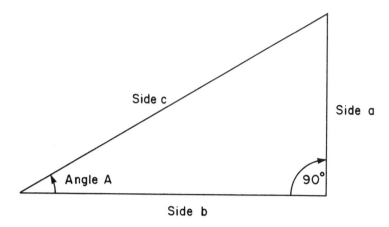

Figure C.1. Sides and angles of a right triangle.

$$\sin A = \tfrac{1}{2} = 0.50$$

$$\cos A = \frac{\sqrt{3}}{2} = 0.87$$

If the sine or cosine is known, angle A may be found using a calculator or a table such as Table C.1.

Example C.2.2

If sin A is 0.5, what is A? From Table C.1, A = 30 degrees.

Example C.2.3

If cos A is 0.87, what is A? From Table C.1, A = 30 degrees.

If angle A is known, sin A or cos A may be found using a calculator or a table such as Table C.1.

Example C.2.4

If A = 40 degrees, what are the sin A and cos A? From Table C.1, sin A = 0.64 and cos A = 0.77.

Table C.1
Sines and Cosines for Various Angles

Angle A (degrees)	sin A	cos A
0	0.00	1.00
1	0.02	1.00
2	0.03	1.00
3	0.05	1.00
4	0.07	1.00
5	0.09	1.00
6	0.10	0.99
7	0.12	0.99
8	0.14	0.99
9	0.16	0.99
10	0.17	0.98
20	0.34	0.94
30	0.50	0.87
40	0.64	0.77
50	0.77	0.64
60	0.87	0.50
70	0.94	0.34
80	0.98	0.17
90	1.00	0.00

Exercises

C.2.1 If side a, b, and c in Figure C.1 have lengths of 3, 4, and 5, respectively, sin A is _____ and cos A is _____.

C.2.2 If angle A is 90 degrees, sin A is _____ and cos A is _____.

C.2.3 If sin A is 0.17, angle A is _____ degrees.

C.2.4 If cos A is 0.94, angle A is _____ degrees.

C.3
Decibels

The logarithm (log) to the base 10 of a number is equal to the number of tens that must be multiplied together to result in that number. More generally, it is the power to which 10 must be raised to give a particular number.

Example C.3.1

What is the logarithm of 1000? To obtain 1000, three tens must be multiplied together:

10 x 10 x 10 = 1000

Three tens then yield the logarithm (log) of 1000.

log 1000 = 3

The logarithm of the reciprocal of a number is equal to the negative of the logarithm of the number.

Example C.3.2

What is the logarithm of 0.01?

$$0.01 = \frac{1}{100}$$

$$\log 100 = 2$$
$$\log 0.01 = \log \frac{1}{100} = -2$$

Decibels are quantities that result from taking 10 times the logarithm of the ratio of two powers or intensities.

Example C.3.3

Compare the following two powers in decibels: power one = 1 W; power two = 10 W.

$$10 \log \frac{\text{power one}}{\text{power two}} = 10 \log \frac{1}{10} = 10(-\log 10) = 10(-1) = -10 \text{ dB}$$

Power one is 10 dB less than power two, or power one is 10 dB below power two. Also

$$10 \log \frac{\text{power two}}{\text{power one}} = 10 \log \frac{10}{1}$$
$$= 10 (\log 10) = 10 (1) = 10 \text{ dB}$$

Power two is 10 dB more than power one, or power two is 10 dB above power one.

Example C.3.4

An amplifier has a power output of 100 mW when the input power is 0.1 mW. What is the amplifier gain in decibels?

amplifier gain (dB) $= 10 \log \dfrac{\text{power out}}{\text{power in}}$

$= 10 \log \dfrac{100}{0.1} = 10 \log 1000 = 10(3) = 30 \, \text{dB}$

Example C.3.5

An electric attenuator has a power output of 0.01 mW when the input power is 100 mW. What is the attenuator attenuation in decibels?

attenuator attenuation (dB) $= -10 \log \dfrac{\text{power out}}{\text{power in}}$

$= -10 \log \dfrac{0.01}{100} = -10 \log \dfrac{1}{10,000} = -10(-\log 10,000)$

$= -10(-4) = 40 \, \text{dB}$

The first minus sign is used here to give the attenuation as a positive number. If the minus number had not been used, the "gain" of the attenuator would have been calculated, which would have turned out to be –40 dB. A gain of –40 dB is the same as an attenuation of 40 dB.

Example C.3.6

Compare intensity two with intensity one; intensity one = 10 mW/cm^2; intensity two = 0.01 mW/cm^2.

$10 \log \dfrac{\text{intensity two}}{\text{intensity one}} = 10 \log \dfrac{0.01}{10}$

$= 10 \log \dfrac{1}{1000} = 10(-\log 1000) = 10(-3) = -30 \, \text{dB}$

Intensity two is 30 dB less than or below intensity one.

Example C.3.7

As sound passes through a medium, its intensity at one point is 1 mW/cm^2 and at a point 10 cm farther along is 0.1 mW/cm^2. What are the attenuation and attenuation coefficient? (See Section 2.4.)

$$\text{attenuation (dB)} = -10 \log \frac{\text{intensity at second point}}{\text{intensity at first point}}$$

$$= -10 \log \frac{0.1}{1} = -10 \log \frac{1}{10} = -10(-\log 10)$$

$$= -10(-1) = 10 \text{ dB}$$

See Example C.3.5 for comment on the first minus sign. The attenuation coefficient is the attenuation (dB) divided by the separation between the two points:

$$\text{attenuation coefficient (dB/cm)} = \frac{\text{attenuation (dB)}}{\text{separation (cm)}}$$

$$= \frac{10 \text{ dB}}{10 \text{ cm}} = 1 \text{ dB/cm}$$

Table C.2 lists various values of power or intensity ratio with corresponding decibel values of gain or attenuation.

Some authors always put output or end-of-path values in the numerator of the equation used for calculating decibels. If the numerator value is less than the denominator value (e.g., attenuation) a negative decibel value is calculated. For example, if the input and output powers for an electrical attenuator were 2 W and 1 W, respectively, -3 dB results. That is, this attenuator has -3 dB of gain. In this book, only positive dB values are considered. In the example, the result would be given as 3 dB of attenuation.

Exercises

C.3.1 Give the logarithms of the following numbers:
    a. 10 _____
    b. 0.1 _____
    c. 100 _____
    d. 0.001 _____

C.3.2 One watt is _____ dB below 100 W.

C.3.3 One watt is _____ dB above 100 mW.

C.3.4 If the input power is 1 mW and the output is 10,000 mW, the gain is _____ dB.

C.3.5 If the input power is 1 W and the output is 100 mW, the gain is _____ dB. The attenuation is _____ dB.

C.3.6 If the intensities of traveling sound are 10 mW/cm^2 and 0.1 mW/cm^2 at two points 5 cm apart, the attenuation between the

Table C.2
Decibel Values of Gain or Attenuation for Various Values of Power or
Intensity Ratio*

dB GAIN OR ATTENUATION	Intensity or Power Ratio	
	ATTENUATION	GAIN
1	0.79	1.3
2	0.63	1.6
3	0.50	2.0
4	0.40	2.5
5	0.32	3.2
6	0.25	4.0
7	0.20	5.0
8	0.16	6.3
9	0.13	7.9
10	0.10	10.0
15	0.032	32.0
20	0.01	100.0
25	0.003	320.0
30	0.001	1000.0
35	0.0003	3200.0
40	0.0001	10,000.0
45	0.00003	32,000.0
50	0.00001	100,000.0
60	0.000001	1,000,000.0
70	0.0000001	10,000,000.0
80	0.00000001	100,000,000.0
90	0.000000001	1,000,000,000.0
100	0.0000000001	10,000,000,000.0

*The ratio is output power or intensity divided by input power or intensity.
In the case of attenuation, it is the fraction of power or intensity remaining.

two points is _____ dB. The attenuation coefficient is _____
dB/cm.

C.3.7 If an amplifier has a gain of 15 dB, the ratio of output power to
input power is _____. (Use Table C.2.)

C.3.8 If an attenuator has an attenuation of 25 dB, the ratio of output
power to input power is _____. (Use Table C.2.)

C.3.9 If the intensity at the start of a path is 3 mW/cm^2 and the attenuation over the path is 2 dB, the intensity at the end of the path is
_____ mW/cm^2. (Use Table C.2.)

C.3.10 If the output of a 22-dB gain amplifier is connected to the input of
a 23-dB gain amplifier, the total gain is _____ dB. The overall
power ratio is _____. (Use Table C.2.)

C.3.11 If a 17-dB attenuator is connected to a 15-dB amplifier, the net
gain is _____ dB. The net attenuation is _____ dB. For a 1-W input,
the output is _____ W. (Use Table C.2.)

C.4
Binary Numbers

The use of digital memories in ultrasound imaging instruments (Section 4.4) presents a need for understanding the binary numbering system. Digital (computer) memories and data processors use binary numbers in carrying out their functions. This is because they contain electronic components that operate in only two states, off (0) and on (1).

Binary digits (bits) consist of only zeros and ones, represented by the symbols 0 and 1. As in the decimal numbering system, with which we are so familiar, other numbers must be represented by moving these symbols to different positions (columns). In the decimal system, where there are ten symbols (0 through 9), there is no symbol for the number ten (nine is the largest number for which there is a symbol). To represent ten in symbolic form, the symbol for one is used but moved to the second (from the right) column. A zero is placed in the right column to clarify this so that ten is, symbolically, 10. The symbols for one and zero have been used but in such a way that they no longer represent one or zero, but, rather, ten.

A similar procedure is used in the binary numbering system. The symbol 1 represents the largest number (one) for which there is a symbol in the system. To represent the next number (two), the same thing is done as in the decimal system. That is, the symbol 1 is placed in the next column to represent the number two.

Columns in the two systems represent values as follows:

decimal: binary:

	millions	hundred-thousands	ten-thousands	thousands	hundreds	tens	ones			sixty-fours	thirty-twos	sixteens	eights	fours	twos	ones

In the decimal system, each column represents ten times the column to the right. In the binary system each column represents two times the column to the right.

The decimal number 1234 represents (reading from right to left) four ones, three tens, two hundreds, and one thousand, i.e., 4 + 30 + 200 +

1000 = 1234. The decimal number 10110 represents zero ones, one ten, one hundred, zero thousands, and one ten thousand. The binary number, 10110, represents zero ones, one two, one four, zero eights, and one sixteen, i.e., $0 + 2 + 4 + 0 + 16 = 22$ (in decimal form). The previous sentence represents a straightforward way of converting a number from binary to decimal. To convert from decimal to binary, repeated division by two is used as follows. Divide the decimal number by two and note the remainder. Divide the quotient (from the previous division) by two and note the remainder. Continue until the quotient is zero. Write the remainders from first to last in order from right to left, respectively, to get the binary number equivalent of the initial decimal number.

Example C.4.1

Convert the decimal number 60 to binary:

		quotient	remainder
2)60	=	30	0
2)30	=	15	0
2)15	=	7	1
2) 7	=	3	1
2) 3	=	1	1
2) 1	=	0	1

The binary form of 60 is, therefore, 111100.

Example C.4.2

Convert the binary number 101010 to decimal form. This number represents $0 + 2 + 0 + 8 + 0 + 32 = 42$ in decimal. To check this answer, convert 42 back to binary.

		quotient	remainder
2)42	=	21	0
2)21	=	10	1
2)10	=	5	0
2) 5	=	2	1
2) 2	=	1	0
2) 1	=	0	1

i.e., 101010.

Table C.3 lists the binary forms of the decimal numbers 0 through 63. Numbers 64 through 127 would have one additional digit, and so forth with higher multiples of 2.

Table C.3
Binary and Decimal Number Equivalents

Decimal	Binary	Decimal	Binary
0	000000	32	100000
1	000001	33	100001
2	000010	34	100010
3	000011	35	100011
4	000100	36	100100
5	000101	37	100101
6	000110	38	100110
7	000111	39	100111
8	001000	40	101000
9	001001	41	101001
10	001010	42	101010
11	001011	43	101011
12	001100	44	101100
13	001101	45	101101
14	001110	46	101110
15	001111	47	101111
16	010000	48	110000
17	010001	49	110001
18	010010	50	110010
19	010011	51	110011
20	010100	52	110100
21	010101	53	110101
22	010110	54	110110
23	010111	55	110111
24	011000	56	111000
25	011001	57	111001
26	011010	58	111010
27	011011	59	111011
28	011100	60	111100
29	011101	61	111101
30	011110	62	111110
31	011111	63	111111

Exercises

C.4.1 In binary numbers, how many symbols are used? _____

C.4.2 The term "binary digit" is commonly shortened into the single word _____.

C.4.3 Each binary digit in a binary number is represented in memory by a memory element, which at any time is in one of _____ states.

C.4.4 Match the following:
Column in a binary number hgfedcba:
a. _____
b. _____
c. _____
d. _____

e. ____

f. ____

g. ____

h. ____

Decimal number represented by a 1 in the column:

1. 64

2. 32

3. 1

4. 16

5. 8

6. 128

7. 2

8. 4

C.4.5 The binary number 10110 represents zero ones, one two, one four, zero eights, and one sixteen, i.e., 0 + 2 + 4 + 0 + 16 = 22. What decimal number is represented by the binary number 11001? ____

C.4.6 The decimal number 13 is made up of one one, zero twos, one four, and one eight (8 + 4 + 0 + 1 = 13). It is therefore represented by the binary number ____.

C.4.7 Match the following:

a. 1 ____	1. 0001111
b. 5 ____	2. 0011001
c. 10 ____	3. 0001010
d. 15 ____	4. 0110010
e. 20 ____	5. 0000001
f. 25 ____	6. 1100100
g. 30 ____	7. 0101000
h. 40 ____	8. 0011110
i. 50 ____	9. 0010100
j. 100 ____	10. 0000101

C.4.8 How many binary digits are required in the binary numbers representing the following numbers?

a. 0 ____

b. 1 ____

c. 5 ____

d. 10 ____

e. 25 ____

f. 30 ____

g. 63 ____

h. 64 ____

i. 75 ____

j. 100 ____

C.4.9 Match the following:
Largest decimal number that can be represented
by a binary number with this many bits

a. 7 _____	1. 1
b. 15 _____	2. 2
c. 3 _____	3. 3
d. 511 _____	4. 4
e. 1023 _____	5. 5
f. 63 _____	6. 6
g. 255 _____	7. 7
h. 1 _____	8. 8
i. 127 _____	9. 9
j. 31 _____	10. 10

C.4.10 How many bits are required to store numbers representing each number of different gray shades?

a. 2 _____
b. 4 _____
c. 8 _____
d. 15 _____
e. 16 _____
f. 25 _____
g. 32 _____
h. 64 _____
i. 65 _____
j. 128 _____

C.5
Units

Units for the physics and acoustics quantities discussed in this book are presented in this section. They are drawn primarily from the international system of units (SI).

Units for the quantities discussed in this book are listed in Table C.4. Equivalent units are given in Table C.5. Prefixes for units are listed in Table C.6, and conversion factors between common units are in Table C.7.

In algebraic equations involving these units, the units for the quantity solved for are determined by manipulation of the units for the other quantities in the equation.

Table C.4
Units and Unit Symbols for Physics and Acoustic Quantities

Quantity	Unit	Unit Symbol or Abbreviation
Acceleration	meters/second^2	m/s^2
Angle	degrees	—
Area	meters^2	m^2
Attenuation	decibels	dB
Attenuation coefficient	decibels/meter	dB/m
Beam area	meters^2	m^2
Current	amperes	A
Density	kilograms/meter^3	kg/m^3
Displacement	meters	m
Doppler shift	hertz	Hz
Energy	joules	J
Force	newtons	N
Frequency	hertz	Hz
Gain	decibels	dB
Half-intensity depth	meters	m
Heat	joules	J
Impedance	rayls	—
Intensity	watts/meters^2	W/m^2
Mass	kilograms	kg
Period	seconds	s
Power	watts	W
Pressure	newtons/meter^2	N/m^2
Propagation speed	meters/second	m/s
Pulse duration	seconds	s
Pulse repetition frequency	hertz	Hz
Pulse repetition period	seconds	s
Resistance	ohms	Ω
Spatial pulse length	meters	m
Speed	meters/second	m/s
Stiffness	newtons/meter^2	N/m^2
Temperature	degrees kelvin	°K
Time	seconds	s
Velocity	meters/second	m/s
Voltage	volts	V
Volume	meters^3	m^3
Wavelength	meters	m
Work	joules	J

Table C.5
Equivalent Units for Physics and Acoustics Quantities

Unit given in Table C.4	Equivalent Unit	Equivalent Unit Abbreviation
Hertz	1/second	1/s
Joules	newton-meters	N-m
Joules	watt-seconds	W-s
Rayls	kilograms/meter^2-second	kg/m^2-s
Newtons	kilogram-meters/second^2	kg-m/s^2
Newtons/meter	pascals	Pa
Watts	joules/second	J/s

Table C.6
Unit Prefixes

Prefix	Factor*	Symbol or Abbreviation
mega	1,000,000	M
kilo	1000	k
centi	0.01	c
milli	0.001	m
micro	0.000001	μ

*Factor is the number of unprefixed units in a unit with the prefix. For example, there are 1000 Hz in 1 kHz, and there is 0.001 m in 1 mm.

Table C.7
Conversion Factors among Common Units

To convert	from	to	multiply by
Area	m^2	cm^2	10,000
	cm^2	m^2	0.0001
Displacement	m	mm	1,000
	m	cm	100
	m	km	0.001
	mm	m	0.001
	mm	km	0.000001
	km	mm	1,000,000
Frequency	Hz	kHz	0.001
	Hz	MHz	0.000001
	kHz	MHz	0.001
	MHz	kHz	1000
	kHz	Hz	1000
	MHz	Hz	1,000,000
Intensity	W/cm^2	W/m^2	10,000
	W/cm^2	kW/m^2	10
	W/cm^2	mW/cm^2	1000
	W/m^2	W/cm^2	0.0001
	W/m^2	mW/cm^2	0.1
	W/m^2	kW/m^2	0.001
Speed	m/s	km/s	0.001
	km/s	m/s	1,000
	km/s	mm/μs	1

Example C.5.1

Determine the unit for frequency in the equation

$$\text{frequency} = \frac{\text{propagation speed (m/s)}}{\text{wavelength (m)}}$$

The units on the right-hand side of the equation are

$$\frac{m/s}{m} = 1/s$$

From Table C.5, it can be found that

$$1/s = Hz$$

Therefore, the frequency unit is hertz.

Example C.5.2

Determine the unit for frequency in the equation

$$frequency = \frac{propagation\ speed\ (m/s)}{wavelength\ (mm)}$$

The units on the right-hand side of the equation are

$$\frac{m/s}{mm}$$

From Table C.6, it can be found that 1 mm equals 0.001 m, so that

$$\frac{m/s}{0.001\ m} = 1000\ 1/s$$

and from Tables C.5 and C.6,

$$1000\ 1/s = 1000\ Hz = 1\ kHz$$

Therefore, the frequency unit is kilohertz. To convert a frequency given in kilohertz to megahertz, multiply by 0.001. To convert a frequency given in kilohertz to hertz, multiply by 1000.

Example C.5.3

Determine the unit for intensity in the equation

$$intensity = \frac{power\ (W)}{area\ (cm^2)}$$

The units on the right-hand side of the equation are

$$\frac{W}{cm^2}$$

Therefore, the intensity unit is watts per centimeter squared.

Example C.5.4

Determine the unit for impedance in the equation

$$\text{impedance} = \text{density (kg/m}^3) \times \text{propagation speed (km/s)}$$

The units on the right-hand side of the equation are

$$\frac{\text{kg}}{\text{m}^3} \times \frac{\text{km}}{\text{s}}$$

From Table C.6,

$$\frac{\text{kg}}{\text{m}^3} \times \frac{\text{km}}{\text{s}} = \frac{\text{kg}}{\text{m}^3} \times \frac{1000 \text{ m}}{\text{s}} = 1000 \frac{\text{kg}}{\text{m}^2\text{-s}}$$

From Table C.5,

$$1000 \frac{\text{kg}}{\text{m}^2\text{-s}} = 1000 \text{ rayls}$$

From Table C.6,

$$1000 \text{ rayls} = 1 \text{ krayl}$$

Therefore, the impedance unit is kilorayl. Since this is uncommon, it would be better to keep the result in rayls.

Exercises

C.5.1 The unit of frequency in the equation

$$\text{frequency} = \frac{\text{propagation speed (km/s)}}{\text{wavelength (mm)}}$$

is _____ . To convert frequency in this unit to frequency in kilohertz, multiply by _____ .

C.5.2 A frequency of 50 kHz is equal to _____ MHz and _____ Hz.

C.5.3 A speed of 1.5 mm/μs is equal to _____ km/s, _____ m/s, _____ cm/s, and _____ mm/s.

C.5.4 If the frequency is 2 MHz and

$$period = \frac{1}{frequency}$$

the period is _____ μs, _____ ms, or _____ s.

C.5.5 Mass is given in units of
a. megahertz
b. kilogram
c. degree kelvin
d. watt
e. none of the above

C.5.6 Displacement is given in
a. megahertz
b. decibel
c. ohm
d. meter
e. all of the above

C.5.7 Attenuation is given in
a. decirayl
b. deciwatt
c. decibel
d. decimeter
e. decihertz

Appendix D
Physics

The terms discussed in this appendix are defined in the Glossary. Their units are given in Appendix C. The definitions are amplified here and the terms are related to one another.

D.1
Mechanics

If there were no forces, everything would be in a state of rest or steady motion. Forces change the state of rest or motion of matter. When considering sound, the force divided by the area over which the force is applied is a useful quantity. This is called pressure, one of the acoustic variables discussed in Chapter 2. It is force per unit area (the concentration of force).

pressure $(N/m^2) = \dfrac{\text{force (N)}}{\text{area (m}^2)}$	$p = \dfrac{F}{A}$

A given force applied to an object may produce markedly different results if the pressures at which it is applied are different. If, for example, a small force is applied by a hand to an inflated toy balloon, the balloon will simply move. If the same small force is applied by a sharp needle, the balloon will break. The difference is that the needle applies the force over a very small area (a very high pressure), breaking the balloon.

Application of force or pressure changes the state of rest or motion of matter. Motion may be described in many ways.

Displacement is the distance that a body has moved.

Speed is the rate at which position is changing. It is the distance moved divided by the time over which the movement occurs.

speed (m/s) = $\dfrac{\text{displacement (m)}}{\text{time (s)}}$	$s = \dfrac{d}{t}$

Velocity is the same as speed except that the direction of motion is specified.

Acceleration is the rate at which velocity is changing. It is the change in velocity (change in speed or direction or both) divided by the time over which the change occurs.

acceleration (m/s^2) = $\dfrac{\text{velocity change (m/s)}}{\text{time (s)}}$	$a = \dfrac{\Delta v}{t}$

Mass is a measure of an object's resistance to acceleration. Weight is the gravitational force between two bodies attracting each other. The mass of a body is the same whether it is on the earth or on the moon, but the weights of the body in the two places are quite different.

Density is the concentration of mass. It is the mass divided by the volume taken up by the mass (mass per unit volume).

density (kg/m^3) = $\dfrac{\text{mass (kg)}}{\text{volume (m}^3\text{)}}$	$\rho = \dfrac{m}{v}$

Stiffness is a description of the resistance of a material to compression. It is equal to the applied pressure divided by the fractional change in volume resulting from the pressure.

stiffness (N/m^2) = $\dfrac{\text{pressure (N/m}^2\text{)}}{\text{fractional volume change}}$	$M = \dfrac{p}{\Delta V_F}$

The fractional volume change is the difference in volume before and after the pressure is applied, divided by the volume before the pressure is applied.

If a material has high stiffness, little change in volume will occur when pressure is applied. If it has low stiffness, a large change in volume will occur when pressure is applied. Stiffness is also called bulk modulus of elasticity. It is equal to one divided by the compressibility of a material.

Newton's second law of motion relates three of the physical phenomena discussed in this appendix. It states that the force applied to a body is equal to the mass of the body multiplied by the acceleration of the body resulting from the applied force.

force (N) = mass (kg) $\times$ acceleration (m/s^2)	F = ma

If more than one force is applied, the net force (resulting from combination of the applied forces) is the force used in the equation. The acceleration will always be in the direction of the net force.

Exercises

D.1.1 To convert speed to velocity, _____ must be specified.

D.1.2 Increased mass results in _____ weight.

D.1.3 Pressure is the concentration of _____.

D.1.4 Density is the concentration of _____.

D.1.5 Speed is the rate at which _____ changes.

D.1.6 Acceleration is the rate at which _____ changes.

D.1.7 Newton's second law of motion states that _____ equals _____ times _____.

D.1.8 Stiffness is a description of the resistance of a material to _____.

D.1.9 If a force of 50 N acts uniformly over an area of 20 m^2, the pressure is _____ N/m^2.

D.1.10 If a body moves 50 m uniformly in 5 s, its speed is _____ m/s.

D.1.11 If a body accelerates uniformly to the east at 5 m/s^2, its velocity 5 s after starting from zero speed is _____ m/s east.

D.1.12 Five kilograms of matter with a volume of 10 m^3 has a density of _____ kg/m^3.

D.1.13 If a pressure of 5 N/m^2 changes the volume of a body from 0.5 m^3 to 0.4 m^3, the fractional volume change is _____.

D.1.14 The stiffness of the material of the body in Exercise D.1.13. is
_____ N/m^2.

D.1.15 A 5-kg mass subjected to a 15-N force west will have acceleration of _____ m/s^2 in the _____ direction.

D.2
Energy

Work is done when a force acts against a resistance to produce motion of a body. It is equal to the applied net force multiplied by the distance the body moves (displacement).

work (J) = force (N) x displacement (m)	W = Fd

If there is no motion, no work is done. If a body is in motion but no force
is being applied, no work is done.

Energy is the capability of doing work. A body must have energy in
order to do work on another body. When a body does work, it loses
energy. When a body has work done on it, it receives energy. Work may
be thought of as the transfer of energy from one body (the one doing the
work) to another (the one having work done on it). The energy transferred is equal to the work done.

Power is the rate at which work is done or the rate at which energy
is transferred. It is equal to the work done divided by the time required
to do the work. It is also equal to energy transferred divided by the time
required to transfer the energy.

power (W) = $\dfrac{\text{work (J)}}{\text{time (s)}} = \dfrac{\text{energy (J)}}{\text{time (s)}}$	$P = \dfrac{W}{t} = \dfrac{E}{t}$

Heat is one type of energy. It is the energy resulting from thermal
molecular motion.

Temperature is the condition of a body that determines transfer of
heat to or from other bodies. No heat flows when two bodies of equal
temperatures come in contact with each other. Heat flows from a body of
higher temperature to one of lower temperature when they come in contact.

Electricity is another type of energy. It is the energy resulting from the displacement or flow of electrons. Electric voltage is the work done when moving a unit electric charge between two points across which the voltage exists. It is measured in volts. Electric current is the rate of flow of electrons in an electric conductor. This flow is caused by a voltage. Electric current is measured in amperes. The quantity of current is determined not only by the voltage but also by the electric resistance of the conductor. Ohm's law relates voltage, current, and resistance.

voltage (V) = current (A) x resistance (Ω)	$V = IR$

Electric power is equal to voltage multiplied by current.

power (W) = voltage (V) x current (A)	$P = VI$

Combining Ohm's law and the electric power equation yields:

power (W) = current^2 (A^2) x resistance (Ω)	$P = I^2 R$
$= \dfrac{\text{voltage}^2 \ (V^2)}{\text{resistance } (\Omega)}$	$= \dfrac{V^2}{R}$

Exercises

D.2.1 Match the following:
   a. pressure: _____
   b. speed: _____
   c. acceleration: _____
   d. density: _____
   e. force: _____
   f. stiffness: _____
   g. work: _____
   h. power: _____
   i. electric power: _____
   j. voltage: _____

1. force x displacement
2. displacement/time
3. mass x acceleration
4. work/time
5. force/area
6. velocity change/time
7. mass/volume
8. pressure/fractional volume change
9. current x resistance
10. voltage x current

D.2.2 Power is the rate at which _____ is done.

D.2.3 Energy is the capability of doing _____.

D.2.4 Temperature is the condition of a body that determines transfer of _____ to or from other bodies.

D.2.5 Heat and electricity are two types of _____.

D.2.6 If the current is 2 amperes and the resistance is 12 ohms, the voltage is _____ V and the power is _____ W.

D.2.7 If the current is 25 mA and the resistance is 50 kΩ, the voltage is _____ V and the power is _____ W.

D.2.8 If current is doubled (constant resistance), voltage is _____ and power is _____.

D.2.9 If resistance is doubled (constant current), voltage is _____ and power is _____.

D.2.10 Ohm's law relates _____ , _____ , and _____.

D.2.11 Voltage times current equals electric _____.

D.2.12 Electric power equals (three correct answers)

   a. current x resistance
   b. current x voltage
   c. voltage x resistance
   d. current^2 x resistance
   e. voltage^2/resistance

D.2.13 For 10 volts and 5 amperes, the power is _____ W.

D.2.14 For 10 ohms and 5 amperes, the voltage is _____ V.

D.2.15 If a force of 3 N moves a body 4 m, the work done is _____ J.

D.2.16 If the movement in Exercise D.2.15. occurs in 6 s, the power is _____ J/s or _____ W.

D.2.17 In Exercise D.2.15, the energy transferred is _____ J.

Appendix E
Comprehensive Multiple-Choice Exam

This examination should take less than two hours to complete (averaging less than one minute per question). The answers are found on pages 344 to 349.

1. Which of the following frequencies is in the ultrasound range?
   a. 15 Hz
   b. 15 kHz
   c. 15 MHz
   d. 17,000 Hz
   e. 17 km
2. The average propagation speed in soft tissues is
   a. 1.54 mm/μs
   b. 0.501 m/s
   c. 1540 dB/cm
   d. 37.0 km/min
   e. 2 to 10 MHz
3. Pulse duration is the _____ for a pulse to occur.
   a. space
   b. time
   c. delay
   d. pressure
   e. reciprocal

4. Spatial pulse length equals the number of cycles in the pulse times
   a. period
   b. impedance
   c. beam width
   d. resolution
   e. wavelength
5. If pulse duration is 1 µs and pulse repetition period is 100 µs, duty factor is
   a. 1 per cent
   b. 10 per cent
   c. 50 per cent
   d. 90 per cent
   e. 100 per cent
6. Which of the following has a significant dependence on frequency in soft tissues?
   a. propagation speed
   b. density
   c. stiffness
   d. attenuation
   e. impedance
7. The attenuation of 5 MHz ultrasound in 4 cm of soft tissue is
   a. 5 dB/cm
   b. 10 dB
   c. 2.5 MHz/cm
   d. 2 cm
   e. 5 dB/MHz
8. If the maximum value of an acoustic variable in a sound wave is 10 units and the normal (no sound) value is 7 units, the amplitude is _____ units.
   a. 1
   b. 3
   c. 7
   d. 10
   e. 17
9. Impedance equals propagation speed times
   a. density
   b. stiffness
   c. frequency
   d. attenuation
   e. path length
10. Which of the following cannot be determined from the others?
    a. frequency
    b. amplitude
    c. intensity

d. power
e. beam area
11. For perpendicular incidence, in medium one, density = 1 and propagation speed = 3 and in medium two, density = 1.5 and propagation speed = 2. What is the intensity reflection coefficient?
   a. 0
   b. 1
   c. 2
   d. 3
   e. 4
12. For perpendicular incidence, if the intensity transmission coefficient is 96 per cent, what is the intensity reflection coefficient?
   a. 2 per cent
   b. 4 per cent
   c. 6 per cent
   d. 8 per cent
   e. 10 per cent
13. The quantitative presentation of frequencies contained in echoes is called
   a. preamplification
   b. digitizing
   c. optical encoding
   d. spectral analysis
   e. all of the above
14. For oblique incidence and medium-two speed equal to twice medium-one speed, the transmission angle will be about _____ times the incidence angle.
   a. ½
   b. 17
   c. 2
   d. 4
   e. 5
15. The range equation describes the relationship of
   a. reflector distance, propagation time, and sound speed
   b. distance, propagation time, and reflection coefficient
   c. number of cows and sheep on a ranch
   d. propagation time, sound speed, and transducer frequency
   e. dynamic range and system sensitivity
16. Axial resolution in a system equals
   a. four times the spatial pulse length
   b. ratio of reflector size to transducer frequency
   c. maximum reflector separation expected to be displayed
   d. minimum reflector separation expected to be displayed
   e. spatial pulse length

17. The doppler frequency shift is caused by
    a. relative motion between the transducer and the reflector
    b. patient shivering in a cool room
    c. a high transducer frequency and real-time scanner
    d. small reflectors in the transducer beam
    e. changing transducer thickness

18. A small (relative to the transducer wavelength) reflector is said to
    _____ an incident sound beam.
    a. focus
    b. speculate
    c. scatter
    d. shatter
    e. amplify

19. In soft tissue, two boundaries that generate reflections are separated
    in axial distance (depth) by 1 mm. With a two-cycle pulse of
    ultrasound the minimum frequency that will axially resolve these
    boundaries is
    a. 1.0 MHz
    b. 2.0 MHz
    c. 3.0 MHz
    d. 4.0 MHz
    e. 5.0 MHz

20. The frequency of an ultrasound transducer is determined primarily
    by which of the following:
    a. element diameter
    b. element thickness
    c. speed of sound in tissue
    d. voltage applied
    e. all of the above

21. The fundamental operating principle of medical ultrasound
    transducers is
    a. Snell's law
    b. Doppler's law
    c. magnetostrictive effect
    d. piezoelectric effect
    e. impedance effect

22. Transducers operating properly in pulse-echo imaging systems
    have a quality factor of approximately
    a. 2–3
    b. 7–10
    c. 25–50
    d. 100
    e. 500

23. The axial resolution of a transducer is determined primarily by the
    a. spatial pulse length
    b. the near-field limit
    c. the transducer diameter
    d. the acoustic impedance of tissue
    e. density
24. The lateral resolution of a transducer is determined primarily by the
    a. spatial pulse length
    b. the near-field limit
    c. the transducer diameter
    d. the acoustic impedance of tissue
    e. applied voltage
25. Which of the following quantities varies most with distance from the transducer face?
    a. axial resolution
    b. lateral resolution
    c. frequency
    d. wavelength
    e. period
26. The near-zone length for a 13-mm diameter unfocused 5-MHz circular transducer is greater than that for which of the following 5-MHz transducers with diameters as listed?
    a. 19 mm
    b. 15 mm
    c. 9 mm
    d. depends on impedance
    e. none of the above
27. If the near-zone length of an unfocused transducer 13 mm in diameter extends (in soft tissue) 6 cm from the transducer face, at which of the following distances from the face can the lateral resolution be improved by focusing the sound from this transducer?
    a. 13 cm
    b. 8 cm
    c. 3 cm
    d. 9 cm
    e. none of the above
28. The lateral resolution of an ultrasound system depends upon
    a. the transducer diameter
    b. the transducer frequency
    c. the speed of sound in soft tissue
    d. memory and display
    e. all of the above
29. Which of the following is a characteristic of a medium through which sound is propagating?

a. impedance
b. intensity
c. amplitude
d. frequency
e. period

30. Which of the following cannot be determined from the others?
    a. frequency
    b. period
    c. amplitude
    d. wavelength
    e. propagation speed

31. For perpendicular incidence, if the impedances of the two media are the same, there will be no
    a. inflation
    b. reflection
    c. refraction
    d. calibration
    e. b and c

32. What is the transmitted intensity if the incident intensity is 1 and the impedances are 1.00 and 2.64?
    a. 0.2
    b. 0.4
    c. 0.6
    d. 0.8
    e. 1.0

33. Increasing frequency
    a. improves resolution
    b. increases half-intensity depth
    c. increases refraction
    d. a and b
    e. a and c

34. Increasing intensity produced by the transducer
    a. is accomplished by increasing pulser voltage
    b. increases sensitivity of the system
    c. increases probability of biologic effects
    d. all of the above
    e. none of the above

35. Ultrasound bioeffects
    a. do not occur
    b. do not occur with diagnostic instruments
    c. are not confirmed below 100 mW/cm^2 SPTA
    d. b and c
    e. none of the above

36. Diagnostic ultrasound frequency range is:
  a. 2 to 10 mHz
  b. 2 to 10 kHz
  c. 2 to 10 MHz
  d. 3 to 15 kHz
  e. none of the above

37. If propagation speeds of two media are equal, incidence angle equals
  a. reflection angle
  b. transmission angle
  c. doppler angle
  d. a and b
  e. b and c

38. If no reflection occurs at a boundary, it always means that media impedances are equal in the case of
  a. perpendicular incidence
  b. oblique incidence
  c. refraction
  d. a and b
  e. b and c

39. Increasing spatial pulse length
  a. accompanies increased transducer damping
  b. is accompanied by decreased pulse duration
  c. improves axial resolution
  d. all of the above
  e. none of the above

40. Place the media in order of increasing sound propagation speed.
  a. gas, solid, liquid
  b. solid, liquid, gas
  c. gas, liquid, solid
  d. liquid, solid, gas
  e. solid, gas, liquid

41. What is the wavelength of 1-MHz ultrasound in tissue with propagation speed 1540 m/s?
  a. 1×10^6 m
  b. 1.54 mm
  c. 1540 m
  d. 1.54 cm
  e. 0.77 cm

42. What is the spatial pulse length for two cycles of ultrasound of wavelength 2 mm?
  a. 4 cm
  b. 4 mm
  c. 7 mm

    d. 1.5 mm

    e. 3 mm

43. Increased damping produces
    a. increased bandwidth
    b. decreased Q factor
    c. decreased efficiency
    d. all of the above
    e. none of the above

44. The doppler effect is a change in
    a. intensity
    b. wavelength
    c. frequency
    d. all of the above
    e. b and c

45. What determines the lower and upper limits of frequency range useful in diagnostic ultrasound?
    a. resolution and imaging depth
    b. intensity and resolution
    c. intensity and propagation speed
    d. scattering and impedance
    e. impedance and wavelength

46. If no refraction occurs as an oblique sound beam passes through the boundary between two materials, what is unchanged as the boundary is crossed?
    a. impedance
    b. propagation speed
    c. intensity
    d. sound direction
    e. b and d

47. If the spatial average intensity in a beam is 1 W/cm^2 and the transducer is 5 cm^2 in area, what is the total acoustic power?
    a. 1 W
    b. 2 W
    c. 3 W
    d. 4 W
    e. 5 W

48. How does the propagation speed in bone compare to that in soft tissue?
    a. lower
    b. the same
    c. higher
    d. cannot say unless soft tissue is specified
    e. b and c

49. Attenuation along a sound path is a decrease in
a. frequency
b. amplitude
c. intensity
d. b and c
e. impedance

50. Reverberation causes us to think there are reflectors that are too great in
a. impedance
b. attenuation
c. brightness
d. size
e. number

51. Doppler shift is zero when the angle between the sound direction and the movement (flow) direction is _____ degrees.
a. 30
b. 60
c. 90
d. 45
e. none of the above

52. A focused transducer 13 mm in diameter has a lateral resolution at the focus of better than (i.e., smaller than)
a. 26 mm
b. 13 mm
c. 6.5 mm
d. depends on frequency
e. none of the above

53. An important factor in the selection of a transducer for a specific application is the ultrasonic attenuation of tissue. Owing to this attenuation, a 7.5-MHz transducer should generally be used for
a. imaging deep structures
b. imaging shallow structures
c. imaging both deep and shallow structures
d. imaging adult intracranial structures
e. all of the above

54. A real-time scan
a. consists of many frames produced per second
b. depends on how short a time the sonographer takes to make a scan
c. is made only between 8 a.m. and 5 p.m.
d. gives a gray-scale image, where the other scans give only an M-mode display
e. none of the above

55. Which of the following is determined by the pulser in an instrument?
    a. frequency
    b. pulse repetition frequency
    c. length of time required for pulse to reach a specific reflector and return to the instrument
    d. more than one of the above
    e. none of the above
56. The standard United States television scanning format has _____ lines per frame and _____ frames per second.
    a. 625, 25
    b. 512, 512
    c. 512, 640
    d. 525, 30
    e. 625, 30
57. In an ultrasound imaging instrument a cathode ray tube is used as a
    a. pulser
    b. receiver
    c. memory
    d. display
    e. scan convector
58. If the power at the output of an amplifier is 1000 times the power at the input, the gain is
    a. 60 dB
    b. 30 dB
    c. 1000 dB
    d. 1000 volts
    e. none of the above
59. The dynamic range of an ultrasound system is defined as
    a. the speed with which ultrasound examination can be performed
    b. the range over which the transducer can be manipulated
    c. the ratio of the maximum to the minimum intensity that can be displayed
    d. the range of pulser voltages applied to the transducer
    e. none of the above
60. The display will generally have a _____ dynamic range than other portions of the ultrasound instrument.
    a. larger
    b. smaller
61. The compensation (swept gain) control serves to
    a. compensate for machine instability in the warm-up time
    b. compensate for attenuation
    c. compensate for transducer aging and the ambient light in the examining room

    d. decrease patient examination time
    e. none of the above
62. A digital scan converter is a
    a. compressor
    b. receiver
    c. display
    d. computer memory
    e. none of the above
63. The number 30 in binary is
    a. 0110
    b. 1110
    c. 1001
    d. 1111
    e. none of the above
64. An ultrasound instrument that could represent 64 shades of gray
    would require an eight-bit memory.
    a. true
    b. false
65. Mechanical real-time devices may be designed such that
    a. a transducer is "rocked" at the skin surface
    b. a transducer is not moved at all
    c. a transducer is rocked and the beam passed through a liquidpath
    d. a and c
    e. all of the above
66. Phased array systems involve the sequential switching of a small
    group of elements along the array.
    a. true
    b. false
67. Duplex doppler presents:
    a. anatomic (structural) data
    b. physiologic (flow) data
    c. impedance data
    d. more than one of the above
    e. all of the above
68. Doppler shift frequencies are usually in a relatively narrow range
    above 20 kHz.
    a. true
    b. false
69. Enhancement is caused by a
    a. strongly reflecting structure
    b. weakly attenuating structure
    c. strongly attenuating structure
    d. frequency error
    e. propagation speed error

70. For a two-cycle pulse of 5 MHz in soft tissue, the axial resolution is
   a. 0.1 mm
   b. 0.3 mm
   c. 0.5 mm
   d. 0.7 mm
   e. 0.9 mm
71. Post processing is the process of assigning numbers to be placed in memory.
   a. true
   b. false
72. The minimum displayed axial dimension of a reflector is approximately equal to _____.
   a. beam diameter
   b. ½ x beam diameter
   c. 2 x beam diameter
   d. spatial pulse length
   e. ½ x spatial pulse length
   f. 2 x spatial pulse length
73. The minimum displayed lateral dimension of a reflector is approximately equal to _____.
   a. beam diameter
   b. ½ x beam diameter
   c. 2 x beam diameter
   d. spatial pulse length
   e. ½ x pulse length
   f. 2 x spatial pulse length
74. In a digital instrument, echo intensity is represented in memory by
   a. positive charge distribution
   b. a number
   c. electron density of the scan converter writing beam
   d. a and c
   e. all of the above
75. M mode recordings have _____ dimension(s).
   a. two spatial
   b. one spatial and one temporal
   c. one doppler and one temporal
   d. one doppler and one spatial
   e. b and c
76. In a mechanical sector scanner (assuming constant lines per frame) the higher the frame rate, the greater the unambiguously displayed depth.
   a. true
   b. could be true depending on sector angle chosen

    c. false

    d. depends on whether or not it is an annular array

    e. depends on impedance

77. Another name for rejection is

    a. threshold

    b. depth gain compensation

    c. swept gain

    d. compression

    e. demodulation

78. The binary number 01001 is _____ in decimal.

    a. 1

    b. 3

    c. 5

    d. 7

    e. 9

79. A reflector may be missing from the display because of

    a. reverberation

    b. propagation speed error

    c. enhancement

    d. oblique reflection

    e. doppler shift

80. If the propagation speed in a soft-tissue path is 1.60 mm/μs, a diagnostic instrument assumes a propagation speed too _____ and will show reflectors too _____ the transducer.

    a. high, close to

    b. high, far from

    c. low, close to

    d. low, far from

    e. none of the above

81. The reflector information that can be obtained from an M mode display includes

    a. distance and motion pattern

    b. transducer frequency, reflection coefficient, and distance

    c. acoustic impedance, attenuation, and motion pattern

    d. all of the above

    e. none of the above

82. Increasing the gain generally produces the same effect as

    a. decreasing the attenuation

    b. increasing the compression

    c. increasing the rectification

    d. both b and c

    e. all of the above

83. A gray-scale display shows
    a. gray color on a white background
    b. reflections with one brightness level
    c. a white color on a gray background
    d. a range of reflection amplitudes or intensities
    e. none of the above
84. Electric pulses from the pulser are applied to the
    a. pulser
    b. transducer
    c. receiver
    d. display
    e. memory
85. Rectification and smoothing (filtering) are parts of
    a. amplipression
    b. rejection
    c. a and b
    d. compression
    e. demodulation
86. Which of the following is performed in a receiver?
    a. amplification
    b. compensation
    c. compression
    d. demodulation
    e. all of the above
87. Continuous-wave sound is used in
    a. all ultrasound imaging instruments
    b. only bistable instruments
    c. all doppler instruments
    d. some doppler instruments
    e. some Fourier instruments
88. If the gain of an amplifier is reduced by 3 dB and input power is unchanged, the output power of the amplifier is _____ what it was before.
    a. equal to
    b. twice
    c. one half
    d. greater than
    e. none of the above
89. Increasing the pulse repetition frequency
    a. improves resolution
    b. increases maximum depth imaged unambiguously
    c. decreases maximum depth imaged unambiguously
    d. both a and b
    e. both a and c

90. If gain was 30 dB and output power is reduced by one half, the new gain is _____ dB.
   a. 15
   b. 60
   c. 33
   d. 27
   e. none of the above

91. If four shades of gray are shown on a display, each twice the brightness of the preceding one, the brightest shade is _____ times the brightness of the dimmest shade.
   a. 2
   b. 4
   c. 8
   d. 16
   e. 32

92. The dynamic range displayed in Problem 91 is _____ dB.
   a. 100
   b. 9
   c. 5
   d. 2
   e. 0

93. The 100-mm test object measures
   a. resolution
   b. pulse duration
   c. SATA intensity
   d. wavelength
   e. all of the above

94. The following measure acoustic output:
   a. hydrophone
   b. optical encoder
   c. 100-mm test object
   d. all of the above
   e. none of the above

95. Real-time imaging is made possible by
   a. scan converters
   b. mechanically driven transducers
   c. gray-scale display
   d. arrays
   e. both b and d

96. Gain and attenuation are usually given in
   a. dB
   b. dB/cm
   c. cm

    d. cm/dB

    e. none of the above

97. Gray-scale display is made possible by

    a. array transducers

    b. cathode ray storage tubes

    c. scan converters

    d. b and c

    e. all of the above

98. An advantage of continuous-wave doppler over pulsed doppler is

    a. depth information

    b. bidirectional

    c. no aliasing

    d. b and c

    e. all of the above

99. Vertical deflections of the display spot are produced by reflections in

    a. the B mode

    b. the B scan

    c. the M mode

    d. the A mode

    e. none of the above

100. In doppler color-flow instruments, color represents

    a. sign (+ or –) of doppler shift

    b. flow direction

    c. magnitude of the doppler shift

    d. amplitude of the doppler shift

    e. a and b

101. Attenuation is corrected for by

    a. demodulation

    b. desegregation

    c. decompression

    d. compensation

    e. remuneration

102. What must be known in order to calculate distance to a reflector?

    a. attenuation, speed, density

    b. attenuation, impedance

    c. attenuation, absorption

    d. travel time, speed

    e. density, speed

103. Which of the following improve sound transmission from the transducer element into the tissue?

    a. matching layer

    b. doppler effect

    c. damping material

    d. coupling medium

    e. a and d

104. Lateral resolution is improved by

    a. damping

    b. pulsing

    c. focusing

    d. reflecting

    e. absorbing

105. Voltage pulses occur at the output of the

    a. pulser

    b. transducer

    c. receiver

    d. display

    e. a, b, and c

106. The doppler effect for a scatterer moving toward the sound source causes the scattered sound (compared to the incident sound) received by the transducer to have

    a. increased intensity

    b. decreased intensity

    c. increased impedance

    d. increased frequency

    e. decreased impedance

107. Axial resolution is improved by

    a. damping

    b. pulsing

    c. focusing

    d. reflecting

    e. absorbing

108. Which of the following are or can be dynamic (real-time)?

    a. A mode

    b. B scan

    c. M mode

    d. all of the above

    e. none of the above

109. Duplex doppler instruments include _____.

    a. pulsed doppler

    b. continuous-wave doppler

    c. B-scan imaging

    d. dynamic imaging

    e. more than one of the above

110. If the doppler shifts from normal and stenotic carotid arteries are 4 kHz and 10 kHz, respectively, for which will there be a problem with a pulse repetition frequency of 7 kHz?

    a. normal

b. stenotic

c. both

d. neither

111. The receiver in a doppler system compares the _____ of the voltage generator and the voltage from the receiving transducer.

a. wavelength

b. intensity

c. impedance

d. frequency

e. all of the above

112. A digital imaging instrument divides the cross-sectional image into

_____.

a. frequencies

b. bits

c. pixels

d. binaries

e. wavelengths

113. Which of the following produce(s) a sector-scan format?

a. rotating mechanical real-time transducer

b. oscillating mechanical real-time transducer

c. phased array

d. oscillating mirror

e. all of the above

114. The piezoelectric effect describes how _____ is converted into _____ by a _____.

a. electricity, an image, display

b. incident sound, reflected sound, boundary

c. ultrasound, electricity, transducer

d. ultrasound, heat, tissue

e. none of the above

115. Propagation speed in soft tissues

a. is directly proportional to frequency

b. is inversely proportional to frequency

c. is directly proportional to intensity

d. is inversely proportional to intensity

e. none of the above

116. The frequencies used in diagnostic ultrasound imaging

a. are much lower than those used in doppler measurements

b. determine imaging depth in tissue

c. determine imaging resolution

d. all of the above

e. b and c

117. As frequency is increased

a. wavelength increases

b. a three-cycle ultrasound pulse decreases in length
c. imaging depth decreases
d. propagation speed decreases
e. b and c
118. In the doppler equation

$$f_D = \frac{2\ fv\ \cos\theta}{c - v\cos\theta}$$

which can normally be ignored?
a. v in the denominator
b. v in the numerator
c. f
d. f_D
e. b and c
119. For which of the following is the reflected frequency less than the incident frequency?
a. advancing flow
b. receding flow
c. perpendicular flow
d. laminar flow
e. all of the above
120. Focusing
a. improves lateral resolution
b. improves axial resolution
c. increases beam width in the focal region
d. shortens pulse length
e. increases duty factor

Comprehensive Examination Answers

Following each answer is the section number in which the subject is discussed. Some answers also have explanatory comments.

1. c. 2.2. Ultrasound is sound of frequency greater than 20 kHz (0.02 MHz). Answer e is not in frequency units.
2. a. 2.2. Propagation speeds in soft tissues are in the range of about 1.4 to 1.6 mm/μs. Answers c and e are not in speed units.
3. b. 2.3
4. e. 2.3. The wavelength is the length of each cycle in a pulse.
5. a. 2.3. Duty factor is pulse duration divided by pulse repetition period.
6. d. 2.4. Propagation speed and impedance increase only slightly with frequency.

7. b. 2.4. The attenuation coefficient of 5-MHz ultrasound is approximately 2.5 dB/cm. The attenuation coefficient times the path length yields the attenuation in dB. Only answer b is given in attenuation (dB) units.

8. b. 2.4. Amplitude is the maximum amount that an acoustic variable varies from the normal value. In this case, 10 minus 7 units.

9. a. 2.2. This is the characteristic impedance.

10. a. 2.4. Amplitude, intensity, power, and beam area are all related to each other. If two of these are known, the others can be found. Frequency is independent of these. All four of them can be known and yet frequency undetermined.

11. a. 2.5. Impedance 1 equals 3 equals impedance 2; thus, there is no reflection.

12. b. 2.5. If 96 per cent of the intensity is transmitted, 4 per cent was reflected. (What is not reflected is transmitted, i.e., the two must add up to 100 per cent.)

13. d. 3.2 and 6.3. Spectral comes from "spectrum," referring to color spectrum. A prism is an optical spectrum analyzer that breaks down white light into its component colors.

14. c. 2.5. If the second speed is twice the first speed, then the transmission angle is twice the incidence angle.

15. a. 2.5. Reflector distance equals one half x speed x time.

16. d. 3.5. If reflectors are separated by less than the axial resolution, they are not separated on the display.

17. a. 6.2.

18. c. 2.5. Scattering occurs with rough surfaces and with heterogeneous media (made up of small particles relative to the wavelength). Large flat surfaces produce specular reflections.

19. b. 3.5. Axial resolution is equal to one half spatial pulse length. Spatial pulse length is equal to the number of cycles in the pulse times wavelength. Wavelength is equal to propagation speed divided by frequency. For 1 MHz, wavelength is 1.54 mm, spatial pulse length is 2 x 1.54, and axial resolution is 1.54 mm, so that two reflectors separated by 1 mm would not be resolved. For 2 MHz, the resolution is 0.77 and the reflectors will be resolved.

20. b. 3.2. The operating frequency of a transducer is such that its thickness is equal to one half the wavelength in the transducer element material.

21. d. 3.2. Transducer elements expand and contract when a voltage is applied, and, conversely, when returning echoes apply pressure to the element, a voltage is generated.

22. a. 3.2. For highly damped transducers, the quality factor (Q) is approximately equal to the number of cycles in the pulse.

23. a. 3.5. Axial resolution is equal to one half spatial pulse length.

24. c. 3.5. Lateral resolution is equal to beam width. Near-zone length is dependent on transducer diameter and, thus, so is the lateral resolution at any given distance from the transducer.

25. b. 3.5. Beam width changes with distance from transducer and, thus, also lateral resolution.

26. c. 3.3. Near-zone length increases with transducer diameter so that the only transducer that would have a shorter near-zone length would be a transducer of smaller diameter.

27. c. 3.3. Focusing can only be accomplished in the near zone of a beam.

28. e. 3.5. Answers a, b, and c all affect the beam. Resolution of the system is also affected by the electronics of the instrument.

29. a. 2.2. All the others are characteristics of the sound.

30. c. 2.2. Frequency, period, wavelength, and propagation speed are all related to each other. However, all four of these can be known and yet the amplitude be undetermined.

31. e. 2.5. For perpendicular incidence there is no refraction. For equal impedances there is no reflection.

32. d. 2.5

$$IRC = \left[\frac{2.64 - 1.00}{2.64 + 1.00} \right]^2 = \left[\frac{1.64}{3.64} \right]^2 = (0.45)^2 = 0.2$$

For an intensity reflection coefficient of 0.2 and an incident intensity of one, the reflected intensity is 0.2 and the transmitted intensity is 0.8.

33. a. 3.5, 2.4, and 2.5. Half-intensity depth decreases with increasing frequency and frequency has no effect on refraction.

34. d. 4.2 and 7.4

35. c. 7.4. This is the AIUM statement on in vivo mammalian bioeffects.

36. c. 3.5. Frequencies lower than this range do not provide the needed resolution whereas frequencies greater than this range do not allow for adequate imaging depth for medical purposes.

37. d. 2.5. Incidence angle always equals reflection angle and, for equal propagation speeds, equals transmission angle as well.

38. a. 2.5. For oblique incidence, it is possible to have no reflection even if media impedances are unequal.

39. e. 2.3, 3.2, and 3.5. Increased transducer damping decreases the spatial pulse length. Increasing spatial pulse length is accompanied by increased pulse duration and degraded axial resolution.

40. c. 2.2

41. b. 2.2. Wavelength is equal to propagation speed divided by frequency.

42. b. 2.3. Spatial pulse length is equal to wavelength times the number of cycles in the pulse.

43. d. 3.2

44. e. 6.2. If frequency changes, wavelength changes also.

45. a. 3.5. See answer to Problem 36.

46. e. 2.5. No refraction means that there is no change in sound direction. This is a result of no change in propagation speed (equal propagation speeds on both sides of the boundary).

47. e. 2.4. If there is 1 W in each square centimeter of area, then there are 5 W in 5 cm^2 of area.

48. c. 2.2. Speeds in solids are higher than in liquids. Soft tissue behaves acoustically as a liquid (it is mostly water).

49. d. 2.4

50. e. 5.3. Reverberation adds additional reflectors on the display deeper than the true ones.

51. c. 6.2.

52. c. 3.3. An unfocused 13-mm transducer has a beam width of 6.5 mm at the near-zone length. Focusing would reduce the lateral resolution below this value (improve it).

53. b. 2.4. A 7.5-MHz transducer can image to only a few centimeters in tissue.

54. a. 3.4 and 4.1. The other answers make little sense.

55. b. 4.2

56. d. 4.5

57. d. 4.5

58. b. 4.3 and C.3. For each 10 dB there is a factor of 10 increase in power.

59. c. 4.3

60. b. 4.3

61. b. 4.3

62. d. 4.4

63. e. 4.4 and C.4. Decimal numbers greater than 15 required at least five bits in a binary number. The number 30 in binary is 11110.

64. b. 4.4. 64 shades require a six-bit memory.

65. e. 3.4. In the answer b, the beam can be reflected off an oscillating acoustic mirror (reflector).

66. b. 3.4. This is a description of a linear switched or sequenced array rather than a phased array.

67. d. 6.4. Answers a and b are both correct. Anatomic data are provided by the real-time B scan and physiologic data are provided by the pulsed doppler portion of the instrument.

68. b. 6.2. Physiologic doppler shift frequencies are usually in the audible frequency range.

69. b. 5.4

70. b. 3.5

$$AR = \tfrac{1}{2}SPL = \tfrac{1}{2}n \times \frac{c}{f} = \tfrac{1}{2}(2)\frac{1.54}{5} = 0.3$$

71. b. 4.4. Postprocessing is the assignment of display brightness to numbers coming out of memory.

72. e. 3.5

73. a. 3.5

74. b. 4.4

75. b. 4.5. In M mode, echo depth is displayed as a function of time.

76. c. 5.5. For constant lines per frame a constant number of pulses must be admitted per frame, and the higher the frame rate the greater the pulse repetition frequency. Therefore unambiguously displayed depth would decrease (less time for echoes to return before the next pulse is emitted).

77. a. 4.3

78. e. c. 4. One plus eight equals nine.

79. d. 2.5

80. c. 2.5. The instrument assumes a speed of 1.54 mm/μs. Echoes will arrive sooner because of their higher propagation speed and will be placed closer than they should.

81. a. 4.5

82. a. 2.4 and 4.3. Increasing gain and decreasing attenuation each increase echo intensity.

83. d. 4.4 and 4.5

84. b. 3.2 and 4.2

85. e. 4.3

86. e. 4.3

87. d. 6.3. All imaging instruments and some doppler instruments use pulsed ultrasound.

88. c. 4.3 and C.3. A reduction of 3 dB is a 50 per cent reduction.

89. c. 5.5. Pulse repetition frequency has no effect on resolution.

90. d. 4.3 and C.3. See answer to Problem 88.

91. c. 4.4 and 4.5

92. b. C.3. A factor of 8 is three doublings, i.e., 3 plus 3 plus 3 dB.

93. a. 7.2

94. a. 7.2

95. e. 3.4

96. a. 2.4 and 4.3

97. c. 4.4

98. c. 6.3 and 6.4

99. d. 4.5.

100. e. 6.5

101. d. 4.3

102. d. 2.5. The range equation relates these three quantities.

103. e. 3.2. The matching layer improves sound transmission by reducing the reflection at the transducer-skin boundary. A coupling medium improves it by removing the air layer between the transducer and the skin.

104. c. 3.3

105. e. 3.2, 4.2, and 4.3

106. d. 6.2

107. a. 3.2

108. d. 4.5. All of these modes are updated many times each second.

109. e. 6.4. They include pulsed doppler and dynamic imaging.

110. c. 6.4. Both doppler shifts exceed one half the pulse repetition frequency. The problem will be aliasing.

111. d. 6.3

112. c. 4.4

113. e. 3.4

114. c. 3.2

115. e. 2.2. Propagation speed is independent of frequency and intensity.

116. e. 2.4 and 3.5

117. e. 2.3 and 2.4

118. a. 6.2. Because physiologic speeds are small compared to the speed of sound in tissues.

119. b. 6.2

120. a. 3.3 and 3.5

Answers to Exercises in the Appendixes

Appendix C

C.1.1. $z - y - 2$; b. $y + z - 1$; c. $z/2y$; d. $3yz$; e. 19; f. 3

C.1.2. a. propagation speed/wavelength; b. power/intensity; c. 1/period

C.1.3. 18

C.1.4. Division by zero is what went wrong.
Note that

$$y + x = \tfrac{1}{2}(7y - 3x)$$

yields

$$2(y + x) = 7y - 3x$$

$$2y + 2x = 7y - 3x$$

$$5x = 5y$$

and $x = y$

so that dividing by $y - x$ is dividing by zero (not allowed in algebra).

C.2.1. 0.6, 0.8
C.2.2. 1, 0
C.2.3. 10
C.2.4. 20

C.3.1. a. 1; b. –1; c. 2; d. –3
C.3.2. 20
C.3.3. 10
C.3.4. 40
C.3.5. –10, 10
C.3.6. 20, 4
C.3.7. 32
C.3.8. 0.003
C.3.9. 1.9
C.3.10. 45, 32,000
C.3.11. –2, 2, 0.63

C.4.1. two (0, 1)
C.4.2. bit
C.4.3. two (off, on)
C.4.4. a. 3; b. 7; c. 8; d. 5; e. 4; f. 2; g. 1; h. 6
C.4.5. 25
C.4.6. 1101
C.4.7. a. 5; b. 10; c. 3; d. 1; e. 9; f. 2; g. 8; h. 7; i. 4; j. 6
C.4.8. a. 1 (0); b. 1 (1); c. 3 (101); d. 4 (1010); e. 5 (11001); f. 5 (11110); g. 6 (111111); h. 7 (1000000); i. 7 (1001011); j. 7 (1100100)
C.4.9. a. 3 (111); b. 4 (1111); c. 2 (11); d. 9 (111111111); e. 10 (1111111111); f. 6 (111111); g. 8 (11111111); h. 1 (1); i. 7 (1111111); j. 5 (11111)
C.4.10. a. 1 (0,1); b. 2 (00,01,10,11); c. 3 (000, 001, 010, 011, 100, 101, 110, 111); d. 4; e. 4; f. 5; g. 5; h. 6; i. 7; j. 7

C.5.1. megahertz, 1000

C.5.2. 0.05, 50,000
C.5.3. 1.5, 1500, 150,000, 1,500,000
C.5.4. 0.5, 0.0005, 0.0000005
C.5.5. b
C.5.6. d
C.5.7. c

Appendix D

D.1.1. direction
D.1.2. increased
D.1.3. force
D.1.4. mass
D.1.5. position
D.1.6. velocity
D.1.7. force, mass, acceleration
D.1.8. compression
D.1.9. 2.5
D.1.10. 10
D.1.11. 25
D.1.12. 0.5
D.1.13. 0.2 (pressure is not needed for the calculation)
D.1.14. 25
D.1.15. 3, west

D.2.1. a. 5; b. 2; c. 6; d. 7; e. 3; f. 8; g. 1; h. 4; i. 10; j. 9
D.2.2. work
D.2.3. work
D.2.4. heat
D.2.5. energy
D.2.6. 24, 48
D.2.7. 1250, 31
D.2.8. doubled, quadrupled
D.2.9. doubled, doubled
D.2.10. voltage, current, resistance
D.2.11. power
D.2.12. b, d, e
D.2.13. 50
D.2.14. 50
D.2.15. 12
D.2.16. 2, 2
D.2.17. 12

References

1. Berman, M.C.: Defining the role of the sonographer. Med. Ultrasound, 8:55-60, 1984.
2. Kremkau, F.W.: Education in the physics of diagnostic ultrasound: Is it necessary? Appl. Radiol., 10:112, 1981.
3. Hykes, D., Hedrick, W., and Starchman, D.: Ultrasound Physics and Instrumentation. New York, Churchill Livingstone, 1985.
4. Powis, R., and Powis, W.: A Thinker's Guide to Ultrasonic Imaging. Baltimore, Urban & Schwarzenberg, 1984.
5. Hill, C.: Physical Principles of Medical Ultrasonics. Chichester, England, Ellis Horwood, 1986.
6. McDicken, W.: Diagnostic Ultrasonics: Principles and Use of Instruments. New York, Wiley & Sons, 1981.
7. Hussey, M.: Basic Physics and Technology of Medical Diagnostic Ultrasound. New York, Elsevier, 1985.
8. Wells, P.N.T.: Biomedical Ultrasonics. New York, Academic Press, 1977.
9. Kremkau, F.W.: Ultrasound instrumentation: Physical principles. In Callen, P.W. (ed.): Ultrasonography in Obstetrics and Gynecology. Philadelphia, W.B. Saunders Co., 1982, pp. 313–324.
10. Kremkau, F.W.: Basic principles and biological effects of ultrasound. In Resnick, M.I. and Sanders, R.C.: Ultrasound in Urology. Baltimore, Williams & Wilkins, 1979, pp. 11–24.

11. Edmonds, P.D., and Dunn, F.: Introduction: Physical description of ultrasonic fields. *In* Edmonds, P.D. (ed.): Ultrasonics. Methods of Experimental Physics. Vol. 19. New York, Academic Press, 1981.

12. Goss, S.A., Johnson, R.L., and Dunn, F.: Comprehensive compilation of empirical ultrasonic properties of mammalian tissues. J. Acoust. Soc. Am., 64:423–457, 1978; 68:93–108, 1980.

13. Carson, P.L., Fischella, P.R., and Oughton, T.V.: Ultrasonic power and intensities produced by diagnostic ultrasound equipment. Ultrasound Med. Biol. 3:341–350, 1978.

14. Nyborg, W.L.: Ultrasonic intensities generated by real-time devices. *In* Winsberg, F., and Cooperberg, P.L. (eds.): Clinics in Diagnostic Ultrasound. Vol. 10: Real-time Ultrasonography. New York, Churchill Livingstone, 1982, pp. 15–17.

15. Barnett, S.B., and Kossoff, G.: Ultrasonic exposure in static and real-time echography. Ultrasound Med. Biol. 8:273-276, 1982.

16. American Institute of Ultrasound in Medicine: Acoustical Data for Diagnostic Ultrasound Equipment. Bethesda, MD, American Institute of Ultrasound in Medicine, 1985.

17. Kremkau, F.W., and Taylor, K.J.W.: Artifacts in ultrasound imaging. J. Ultrasound Med. 5:227–237, 1986.

18. Sanders, R.C.: Atlas of Ultrasonographic Artifacts and Variants. Chicago, Year Book Medical Publishers, 1986.

19. Kremkau, F.W.: Seeing and hearing blood flow noninvasively using the doppler shift. Diagn. Imaging, 7:131–133, 1985.

20. Kremkau, F.W.: Technical considerations, equipment, and physics of duplex sonography. In Grant, E.G. and White, E.M.: Duplex Sonography. New York, Springer-Verlag, 1988, pp 1-6.

21. Atkinson, P., and Woodcock, J.P.: Doppler Ultrasound and Its Use in Clinical Measurement. New York, Academic Press, 1982.

22. Goldstein, A.: Quality Assurance in Diagnostic Ultrasound. Bethesda, MD, American Institute of Ultrasound in Medicine, 1980.

23. Banjavic, R.A.: Design and maintenance of a quality assurance program for diagnostic ultrasound equipment. Semin. Ultrasound, 4:10–26, 1983.

24. Kremkau, F.W.: Safety and long-term effects of ultrasound: What to tell your patients. *In* Platt, L.D. (ed.): Perinatal Ultrasound. Clin. Obstet. Gynecol., 27:169–175, 1984.

25. Nyborg, W.L.: Physical mechanisms for biological effects of ultrasound. DHEW publication (FDA) 78-8062. Rockville, MD, U.S. Food and Drug Administration, 1977.

26. American Institute of Ultrasound in Medicine: Bioeffects Considerations for the Safety of Diagnostic Ultrasound. J. Ultrasound Med., 7(Suppl.), 1988.

27. National Council on Radiation Protection and Measurements: Biological Effects of Ultrasound: Mechanisms and Clinical Applications. Bethesda, National Council on Radiation Protection, 1983.
28. Nyborg, W.L., and Ziskin, M.C.: Biological Effects of Ultrasound. New York, Churchill Livingstone, 1985.
29. Williams, A.R.: Ultrasound: Biological Effects and Potential Hazards. New York, Academic Press, 1983.
30. World Health Organization: Environmental Health Criteria 22: Ultrasound. Geneva, World Health Organization, 1982.

Index